LIVE TO 120
WITHOUT SICKNESS AND DISEASE?

LEONARD F. BURNS

May this book serve to enhance your health and prolong your life!

in Jesus Name

LFBurns

CONTENT

FOREWORD

In the United States we tend to take it for granted that when we get old we will develop some form of disease or illness that will ultimately take our lives. It is rare for a person to just die of old age anymore, without succumbing to some dreadful disease that leads to a painful demise. Have you ever wondered why that is so, or why do all people seem to eventually get a disease before they die. Do you think God intended for us to go out in such a fashion, when His Son died that we might live victorious lives? We should leave this life or realm when and only when our assignments are complete and we are ready to die. This would be a dignified and graceful way to leave this earthly realm. This type of death is possible but only experienced by a few. That is a shame because God wants us all to go out that way, but because of our disobedience to the Word of God, we come to the end of our lives in utter despair and agony. Our Standard American Diet, hereafter referred to as SAD, is directly or indirectly responsible for practically all the sickness and disease that ultimately take our lives. The Bible outlines a safe and healthy diet for us. I realize that most people have never read the Bible, however just using common sense, many have figured out what constitutes good wholesome food, yet many more people are daily digging their own graves with their teeth.

In this book we will take a serious look at what we are eating, why we are eating it and what we need to change to experience longevity. There are many people in the world who are living past 100 years and they are doing it disease free. As a matter of fact, there are people in this world who are over 140 years old and still working and maintaining their lives. Our media does not mention these people because if they were featured, Americans would question our short life spans. Why can't you be one of these statistics? You can, but you will never make it eating the junk we Americans eat each and everyday. You would have to make some drastic changes. Remember the old saying, "you are what you eat," that statement has never been truer! Whether you believe in God or not, I do, and therefore I will mention God and His Holy Word, the Bible often in this book. If you can objectively read the Bible, regardless of your spiritual beliefs, you will definitely gain insight that will prolong your life. This book is written for everyone who eats to live and for the many who unfortunately live to eat as well, regardless of their spiritual orientation.

For those of you who consider yourselves members of the Body of Christ, I wonder do you believe Gods' Word? In the Bible God outlines for us what we should eat and what we shouldn't. I personally don't believe God makes suggestions, so what He says, I believe He means. God said that we were designed to eat fruits and vegetables and that the plants we eat were also to be our medicines. Because of Gods grace and mercy, He has allowed us to broaden our choices in foods, but we were designed originally to eat a certain way. To eliminate diseases from our bodies we need to return to Gods' best. The Bible says that "faith comes by hearing," the Word of God. Rom. 10:17 It means you should keep hearing and hearing and hearing, because faith will continue to come. When you stop hearing, faith ceases to come. The Bible also talks about knowing the truth to get set free. John 8:32 We use the word know all the time in our society, yet we really don't know. In the New Testament of the Bible, which was originally written in Greek, the word for know is GINOSKO, and it is interesting to really understand what it means. The word know (Ginosko), means to perceive,

2

resolve and understand to the point where you can thoroughly analyze and distinguish with familiarity. To further break that down, it is saying that you have to experience something to know it. This is why the Bible said that Adam knew Eve and she conceived a child. Gen. 4:1 They experienced each other. The next time someone ask you if you know something, don't be to hasty in replying. Maybe we all should limit our use of the word! The point I am trying to make is this – until we obediently do Gods' Word , we can't know Gods' Word and thereby experience the blessings.

James 1:22-25 (The Amplified Bible)

22. "But be doers of the Word

23. [obey the message], and not merely listeners to it, betraying yourselves [into deception by reasoning contrary to the Truth].

24. For if anyone only listens to the Word without obeying it and being a doer of it, he is like a man who looks carefully at his [own] natural face in a mirror;

25. For he thoughtfully observes himself, and then goes off and promptly forgets what he was like.

26. But he who looks carefully into the faultless law, the [law] of liberty, and is faithful to it and perseveres in looking into it, being not a heedless listener who forgets but an active doer [who obeys], he shall be blessed in his doing (this life of obedience)."

The last point I want to make concerns a scripture found in Rev. 13:17. This scripture talks about the fact that all humanity will receive and be obligated to use a mark to both buy and sell, before this world ,as we know it, ceases. Most people don't realize that the initial framework for this system, concerning the mark, is already in place. Major food conglomerates are also the owners of the major seed companies and they have genetically modified many seeds to receive patents so they can control food production and distribution worldwide. That to me sounds like the groundwork for the system referenced in Revelation 13. Remember "......satan is the prince of this worlds' system." John 14:30

I am an ordained, licensed minister and a former pastor and as such I have been called upon to conduct memorial services. I am tired of conducting funeral services for individuals who actually took themselves out by their dietary choices. These same individuals were members of the Body of Christ, who had been blood bought by Christ' sacrifice and had supposedly offered their bodies as living sacrifices...... Rom. 12:1,2 (Message Bible) "So here's what I want you to do, God helping you: Take your everyday, ordinary life – your sleeping, eating, going-to-work, and walking-around life – and place it before God as an offering, Embracing what God does for you is the best thing you can do for Him. Don't become so well-adjusted to your culture that you fit into it without even thinking. Instead, fix your attention on God. You'll be changed from the inside out. Readily recognize what He wants from you, and quickly respond to it. Unlike the culture around you, always dragging you down to its level of immaturity. God brings the best out of you, develops well-formed maturity in you."
Our love affair with food needs to cease. We should be eating to live and not living to eat. How can God use your temple, when you can't even get up and move properly in response to His commands, because of the effect wrong foods have had on you body?

A great man once said, "ignorance is no longer an adequate excuse for failure, because virtually all limitations are self imposed." Another great writer once said, "it is your responsibility

4

in the final analysis to overcome ignorance. This can only be accomplished if you remain receptive and teachable." This book is dedicated to those who want to make a change, those tired of being sick and tired, those who have tried every diet known to man and for those who have given up hope altogether! I guarantee you that if you will just apply some of this information to your daily regimen, you will see change and live longer. If you apply all of this information, you will be completely transformed and on your way to that 120 years, that we were promised.

If at times you should detect frustration or even anger in my discourse, I apologize in advance. I love you all, however I want this so bad for you that it pains me to see the conditions people are in because of their food choices and trusting natures. Of all the ethnic groups that are represented in America, the African American has the highest rate of practically all the diseases mentioned in this book. Why is that? I don't have any facts to back up the following statement but I do believe that it is true. African Americans are too trusting of the establishment, due in part to their forced obedience, stemming from slavery. That trusting nature has survived several generations and is still influencing them today. I can still hear some of the old folks saying, "yeeaah and he is a doctor, child," and "my doctor said," as if a doctor is God! Many African Americans still view doctors the same way. I personally have just as much respect for doctors as anyone, however I realize that they are practicing medicine and anyone that is practicing anything, can make mistakes and give the wrong advice. The health conditions of the African American is far worst than the health of any other ethnic group in America. I am not blaming doctors for this problem but I am placing the responsibility for their health issues squarely on their own shoulders. This book does not focus on one race only but the information is for all Americans, as it can aid us all in making some healthy decisions concerning food choices. Be blessed by the books contents and invite me to your 120th birthday party!!!

CHAPTER ONE

UNDERSTANDING FOOD
FROM GOD'S PERSPECTIVE

GODS FOOD PLAN

God designed man to live forever because we were made in His image and likeness. God is perfect and when He made man He said that the creation was good. We were made perfect in His sight. Since our bodies were designed for us to live forever, we need to realize that we are continuously recycling cells moment by moment. We are not the same people we were say 10 years ago because our cells are constantly dying or shedding and being renewed. This is why man was able to live for so long initially. Due to sin however, which caused the flood during Noah's day, the earth's atmosphere was drastically changed and the earth was forever altered. Prior to that flood, it had never rained and the earth was a sealed chamber similar to a vacuum or a perfect environment. Sin caused the devastation, which we refer to as the flood, however it had a greater impact on our earth than anyone could have ever imagine and far to catastrophic to just be called a flood. At any rate prior to that flood some species of dinosaurs still existed and men lived to be almost a 1000 years old as evidenced by Methuselah (969 years), who died in the flood. By contrast after the flood, God told Noah that men would live to 120 years. As I stated earlier God planned for man to live forever. These facts are important in understanding God's food plan for man.

Since we have concluded that man was designed to live forever, lets look at the part food would play in this design. If man was to have great longevity, his food would not only have to feed and sustain him but also cure him when necessary. God designed man to be an herbivore initially, look at Gen. 1:29; 2:9, Ezel. 47:12 and Rcv. 22:2. From these scriptures we can get an indication of God's original plan, which clearly indicate that we were to be fully sustained by vegetation. Later because of our rebellion, God allowed us to eat certain meats. His original plan and design for the body however emphasized that we were designed to be vegetarians. If God had intended for us to be carnivores or even omnivores as most of us are, we would have been designed to fully digest flesh. Animals who live on meat have huge incisors, capable of tearing meat apart and they usually go days between meals so that the previous meal can be fully digested. Their digestive systems contain the enzymes and proper acids to fully breakdown the massive amount of protein also. We can eat meat, however we should limit our intake of meat, if we are concerned with longevity. Back to what God said, HE said, our food should also be our medicine. In order for our food to be our medicine, we should primarily be consuming fruits and vegetables, because they can provide all we need. Before I go any further, I want to make it clear that this book is not in anyway an indictment against meat eaters or anyone for that matter. My reason for writing this book is to point out what God's best is and get the Body of Christ to make some changes and take personal responsibility for their health. I will make this statement a lot in this book, I am tired of seeing the Body of Christ suffer and die with the same health issues as the world, when Jesus died that we could be healed and whole. Many times when Jesus healed people He would say, "go and sin no more". Could it be that we are sinning by not listening to the Holy Spirit, taking God's Word too lightly and or putting too much trust in our so called experts? Are we too lazy to find out what causes our problems in the first place, before we let our experts treat the symptoms only? When we do get healed, whether by the doctors or divinely, do we go right back to business as usual and not make changes in our habits? We need to be more responsible and not so lazy. Praying to God is the right thing, but can we help ourselves? God said that we can do all things, with His power and grace. You can't cast out the calories after you have eaten them, not even if you pray it in Jesus name. You can not even bind those pounds in the name of Jesus. These are just two of the prayers that I've heard the saints pray. Many people have asked for prayer concerning their health issues, but they don't want any suggestions or information concerning the things they may or may not be doing to cause the problem. Many times we need to do something or step out in faith or put action to our faith. In the book of 2 Kings, chapter 5, we find the story of Naaman, a army captain who had leprosy. He wanted the man of God to pray that he be healed. The prophet prayed and gave Naaman Gods' instructions, which were to dip himself in the Jordan river seven times. He was first upset with the response because it made no sense but later obeyed and was healed. Many times God will answer peoples' prayers with instructions as to what they should do. Gods' instructions may or may not make sense to you but Just Do It! Is he telling you anything? We will talk more about this dilemma in a later chapter, but as you read this book, ask yourself, is it talking to me? "If you will change your thinking, you will change your life." This is a true statement made by a great American and it is verified in scripture. "...as a man thinketh in his heart, so is he...." Prov. 23:7

From a biblical point of view, God and science are in agreement and from a scientific point of view the Bible is totally verifiable. You may not believe that, however those who have studied both extensively, are aware of this fact. True science, studied by those few enlightened scientist, who have remained teachable and objective, points to the fact that there is a God and He is who He said He is. The world renowned microbiologist, Dr. Robert Young has done pioneering research concerning the PH factor in humans and how a balance PH system is synonymous with divine health. In this book I will not attempt to get too scientific, but I will briefly state what Dr. Young has discovered and you can read his books at your leisure.

Dr. Young clearly understands that God had created man to live indefinitely and provided him with a body that will stay healthy and fight off any ailment if given the opportunity to do so. He found out through his historic studies and research that the PH scale, which is a 14 points scale that measures the ratio of acidity to alkalinity in the body, has a direct correlation to the health condition of all individuals. His studies show that poor diet is linked to an overly acidic body and a healthy body by contrast is balanced at about 7.4, which indicates more alkaline. Before I go any further I will explain to those who may not be familiar with this concept and how the scale works. From 0-6.9 is considered acidic and 7 is neutral, with 7.1-14 being alkaline. Our bodies are designed by God to maintain a healthy PH level, if we eat the proper foods and avoid the bad foods. Our different body systems have different PH levels depending on how the various parts and organs function but there is still a balance that should be maintained. For instance, because our digestive system and intestines are associated with the breakdown and elimination of foods and waste, the PH is more acidic in these areas. Our blood should be at the 7.4 mark and this is important because of the vital work the blood performs in taking nutrients to each cell and oxygenating the system. Our primary concern in this explanation will be the blood. If our systems are highly acidic, we are creating the perfect environment for sickness and disease. If our systems are more alkaline, we tend to not suffer from sicknesses and diseases. A newborn baby, who has had the proper prenatal care will be born in divine health and have a PH factor around the 7.4 mark. A person who is elderly, when they die will have an extremely low level, indicating that the body is totally acidic. This is understandable because a dead body starts decomposing immediately. It is the acidic condition that begins this process. Now we all fall somewhere between these two extremes. The closer you are to the 7.4 mark or slight alkaline state the healthier you will be and on the other hand the more diseases you have will be substantiated by your acidic condition. According to Dr. Young we should eat healthy diets and consume balanced meals in the 80% alkaline/20% acidic range. If we do so and take healthy supplements, he believes we should live well into our 100's or even 200 years.

Before we go to chapter two, I want to explain a few more important concepts that will help you to see how you can live long and strong. We are all born with friendly bacteria in our systems, which lend to the acidity in our systems. The friendly bacteria is in our bodies to help us breakdown, assimilate and utilize food and to dispose of the waste and dead cells which are recycled continuously. When we introduce too much acidic food into our systems it effects the good bacteria in a negative way. The good bacteria can change into yeast (candida) and more acid foods can change the yeast into fungus and still further damage can result when the fungus changes into mold throughout your body. When we talk about these conditions, we are talking about tumors, cancers, diabetes and other chronic health conditions.

Bacteria, yeast (candida), fungus and mold are all types of microforms. According to Dr. Robert Young in his book entitled, "THE PH MIRACLE – Balance Your Diet, Reclaim Your Health," the following list of diseases are attributed to this problem and he makes the following comment. "Most diseases, especially chronic and degenerative ones, follow microform overgrowth. Between the extremes of athlete's feet and AIDS are the yeast and fungus overgrowths underlying symptoms such as diabetes, cancer, atherosclerosis (clogged arteries), osteoporosis, chronic fatigue, and more-including infections that appear to be transmitted person to person. The general signs of overgrowth include pain, infection, fatigue, and body malfunctions including adrenal/thyroid failure, indigestion, diarrhea, food cravings, intestinal pain, depression, hyperactivity, antisocial behavior, asthma, hemorrhoids, colds and flu, respiratory problems, endometriosis, dry skin and itching, thrush, receding gums, finger/toenail fungus, dizziness, joint pain, bad breath, ulcers, colitis, heartburn, dry mouth, PMS and menstrual problems, irritability, puffy eyes, lack of sex drive, skin rash and hives, lupus, mood swings, hormonal imbalance, vaginal yeast infection, cysts and tumors, rheumatoid arthritis, numbness, hay fever, acne, gas/bloating, bowel stasis, low blood sugar, hiatal hernia, headaches, lethargy/laziness, insomnia, suicidal tendencies, coldness/shakiness, infections, over- and underweight conditions, chemical sensitivity, poor memory, muscle aches, allergies (airborne/food), burning eyes, multiple sclerosis, malabsorption, and bladder infections (whew!). And that's not even including that general, just overall bad feeling so common these days. You can blame that on out-of-control miroforms and their toxic acid wastes as well."

Won't you agree that is quite a list. I'm sure you found at least one condition you can identify with. The truth is everyone of these diseases can be stopped and you can walk in divine health but only if you change your thinking, which will result in making better and wiser choices. It is to that end that this book is written. Now let's correct our problems!!

Key points outlined in chapter

(1)

(2)

(3)

(4)

(5)

Changes I can make to improve my health

(1)

(2)

(3)

(4)

(5)

CHAPTER TWO
THE EVOLUTION OF FOOD PRODUCTION

GOD'S INSTRUCTIONS CONCERNING FOOD

During the time of Christ the people enjoyed an agrarian society where food was not only produced locally, but in most cases home grown. Because of this fact, the foods were basic and obviously conducive to the locale they were grown in. This may not seem very important to you, but it was very important to the citizens locally from a standpoint of health. This is very important so I will explain it to you. Because God is our source for all our needs and the creator of life, He sees fit to allow certain foods to grow in certain locations during certain times of the year for our enjoyment and most important for our nutritional sustenance. This fact is crucial to our well being and longevity. In the Garden of Eden God had provided the necessary food products for man to live healthy lives on earth. "And God said,

Behold I have given you every herb bearing seed, which is upon the face of all the earth, and every tree, in the which is the fruit of a tree yielding seed; to you it shall be for meat." (Gen. 1:29) Now these plants had been planted by God and obviously were the right plants for the nourishment of man at that time. God gives us the knowledge and grace to grow our own foods, but His infinite power causes the seeds to reproduce and sustain us and He causes what we call weeds to grow also, which in most cases are great sources of nutrition by themselves. The point is locally grown food is always the freshest and most nutritious food you can eat. In most cases we are not eating locally grown foods. Our food products come from thousands of miles away in many instances. This fact leads to problems, which will be discussed later in this book. You will see as you progress through this book that what God planned and intended, was for the best and we have strayed from Gods' plan and are suffering as a result.

There are several points in the above paragraph that I would like to elaborate on before we continue. The first important point, which I will repeat, is that initially God created man to be a vegetarian. Now before you start throwing rocks at me, let me clarify something. You will see later on in the chapter on Sickness and Disease, that meat-eating plays a bigger role in your overall health problems than first thought but for now track with me. In the beginning God designed a perfect system that we humans failed to adapt to. When man fell in the Garden of Eden by exchanging a perfect world in which God would spiritually direct for an imperfect world controlled by satan and his fear tactics, man forever changed his health condition also.

The second important thing to be gleaned from the first paragraph is the fact that we humans should be eating to live and not living to eat. When you eat to live you eat what is good for you and not necessarily what is good to you because your main objective is to sustain a healthy body for as long as you can. As believers and members of Christ body, we understand that our bodies are His' because He paid dearly for them. (I Cor. 7:23) In the 12th chapter of Rom. Verse 1, we are told that we are to reasonably sacrifice our bodies. Personally my wife and I want to live as long as we can so that we can be a blessing to as many people as God sees fit to send our way. It would be impossible for God to use a person who ate themselves to death or dug their own grave with their teeth. God did say in His Word that we should enjoy the fellowship or covenant meal, just as Jesus did with His disciples, however in our case we get to involved with our foods sometimes. It is possible to make food your God, in which case you would be worshiping an idol. I am only pointing out things or issues we need to be concerned about as believers. We are in this world but not of it as the Word of God said, which means we should operate by Kingdom principles.

Initially mankind would have been classified as hunters and gatherers because they did more foraging for food. As time progressed, more and more of the Israelites began to farm. When they entered the Promised Land, where the land allotments were handed out, they were able to finally settle down and rest from 40 years of nomadic life. At that time, the children of God began to raise their crops. God instructed them concerning how to utilize the land effectively and efficiently. This is a very important point to remember. In the book of Leviticus in the 25th chapter God said that they were to sow their crops for six years then let the land lie dormant in the seventh year. The land was to receive rest during that seventh year. Why did God tell them to do this. Any good farmer knows that the period of rest for the land would allow whatever grew to die and be plowed under so that the nutrients from the dead plants would replenish the soil for the next six years of productive growth. In most industrialize nations, they are not allowing the land to rest because of the potential loss of revenues. The rest is vital to the production of good food and it is also environmentally sound also for the balance of nature and the ecosystem of any area. It has been pointed out by scientist that to restore just the top 1 inch of nutrient rich topsoil to a damaged area could take 1000 years. God also told His people not to sow their fields with mingled seeds. Lev. 19:19. Mingled seeds are hybrid seeds or seeds that has been cross pollinated. When you intentionally modify a plant by scientifically or genetically crossing two different species of plants, it is not good. When plants cross pollinate on their own from pollen transmission caused by birds and bees, God is not concerned. You may ask, why is that a problem? When plants are genetically tampered with , the nutrient value of the plant is compromised. Also hybrid seeds can not reproduce themselves, therefore no fertile seed is produced for the next generation of plants. God is concerned with our nutrition and we should be also. If you are not going to be nourished by your food, then why bother to eat? I am laying the groundwork for your clear understanding of the material to be covered later on in this book.

Food has such a direct correlation with health in the body. This should be an obvious point, however with all the health issues in our society today, it may not be such a no-brainier. The Bible does not have a whole lot to say about food, however it does say some key things. Because we live in a completely different society today than the one our biblical forefathers did, should not excuse us from understanding some vital things concerning our nutrition. God wants us well and there are numerous scriptures to validate this point, but the important question is do we want to be healthy or are we satisfied with a short diseased existence culminating in a horrible death. My family loves good health and we know how to maintain it and we are determined to live long and well before we die a peaceful death.

Concerning meats, when God allowed early man to eat flesh, he was told which animals to eat and which to avoid. The animal stressed most to avoid was the pig. In the book of Leviticus, chapter 11 many animals are outlawed from consumption, including the pig. The pig is to be avoided for numerous reasons. (1) It will eat anything, (2) It does not perspire, so poisons can't escape through any pores and it wallows in anything to keep cool, since it doesn't perspire and (3) Toxins and bacteria do not affect it very much because of its' immune system but these poisons can be passed on to consumers through its' meat. God also said not to eat any flesh that has not been completely drained of blood, because pathogens, toxins and other waste reside in the blood stream. Many of us eat our meats much to rare, to the point of being almost raw.

The bible does mention the following foods to eat:
Fruits & Nuts - apples, almonds, dates, figs, grapes, melons, olives, pistachio nuts, pomegranates, raisins, sycamore fruit
Vegetables & Legumes - beans, cucumbers, gourds, leeks, lentils, onions

Grains – barley, bread, corn, flour, millet, spelt, wheat
Fish

Dairy – butter, cheese, curds, milk

Meats – calf, goat, lamb, oxen, sheep, venison
Fowl – partridge, pigeon, quail, dove

Miscellaneous – eggs, honey, grape juice, locust, wine

In summarizing this section on biblical foods and God's food instructions, we need to review some important things that we have covered which will serve us later as we proceed with our understanding of health in the body. God does not make suggestions. When He tells us things, He expects us to obey because as members of the Body of Christ, we are expected to be obedient. When we are obedient, we won't have to sacrifice. I Sam. 15:22. I believe that just because God is so loving and merciful and we don't visually see His anger, we conclude that it is ok to disobey. The problem with disobedience is that it opens the door for the enemy to attack and we know that the enemy kills, steals and destroys. John 10:10 Has satan tried to attack your body? What door did you open? To the extent we obey, our blessings come and the opposite is also true. To walk in God's best, we need to follow His instructions to the letter. When you do an exhaustive study of God's Word, you will notice that God doesn't continuously mention the consequences for disobedience. This is a fact because He expects you to take Him at His Word and just obey him! If God spent all His time outlining what would occur if you disobeyed, the Bible would be thicker than it is. If you don't believe it look at Deut. 28. God outlines blessings for obedience from verses 1-14, but curses for disobedience are outlined from verses 15-68.

FOOD PRODUCTION FROM SLAVERY TO THE EARLY 1900'S

With the help of slave labor, provided by the unfortunate abduction of a major portion of Africa's population, this country experienced a production boom in both food crops but especially commodities. The small mom and pop farms still provided food for families, but major farms developed during these times started to provide foods and products for entire communities and in some cases towns and cities. As far as food is concerned, the people who had wealth ate well, but those who didn't had to struggled to survive. This of course was evident with the slaves, who learned to basically eat garbage to survive. Slavery has been over now for one hundred and fifty years, yet our soul food diets haven't evolved very much. I mentioned earlier about the health problems in the African American population and much stems from our lack of education concerning health. I believe God directed me to write this book to educate the people. This period of time opened the eyes of the country, especially the farmers, to the concept of mega farms. The major plantations continued to produce up until the war between the states, which was lost by the South, thus ending the slave period. Because commodity crops like cotton and tobacco were very labor intensive, without slave labor many of the plantations folded. However the ones that didn't completely fold switched to share cropping, either with the aid of former slaves or poor whites. It was during this time period that farms focused on food crops to support the families and to sell at market for income. From that period of time up until World War II these farms flourished with bumper crops of produce and good quality food. This is really the beginning of the mega farms which focused on growing produce. As a nation we ate many fruits and vegetables and less meat than we as a nation eat today. I might add that the food was basically organic and the meats contained no hormones , antibiotics nor harmful additives as they do today. Up until this time pesticides, herbicides and antibiotics were foreign terms.

FOOD PRODUCTION CHANGES AFTER THE WAR
Everything changed after the war ended, as far as quality food production was concerned. With war came the industrial revolution and many factories were started to support the war. War is a money making machine in case you did not know that. As long as we are at war, billions of dollars are generated and amassed by a select few. Many people became wealthy and many of the industrialists, their family members and business colleagues became millionaires during this time period. At war's conclusion many of the giant corporations that produced war supplies were stuck with surpluses of various chemicals and substances that they did not know what to do with. These businesses had gotten use to making millions of dollars and they wanted the profits to continue. New businesses sprang up and some of the war surplus products were redirected to the American consumer.

One of the byproducts of war was a chemical used in the atomic bomb, which turned out to be fluoride. This additive was proposed by lobbyist to our government to help fight tooth decay. Fluoride was added to everything possible because of the large surplus left over after the war and we are still dealing with the health issues associated with the use of fluoride in toothpaste, water supplies and elsewhere.

The owners of the ammunition factories convinced the government to use some of the ingredients used in their ammunition as fertilizer to improve the crop yields and food production. As a result another byproduct of war was introduced into the consumer market. What was born was chemical fertilizer, which was suppose to help the farm industry and the government meet demands for cheaper food. The chemical fertilizers, which were suppose to increase production, did so, however they also poisoned the soil, water sheds and upset the balance of the ecosystems in the farm areas. These are just two of the substances that were born during war and utilized later to provide apparent help for the consumer. It is all about money! I hope that you are seeing how our food supply has changed or evolved into what it is today and how our health has declined as a result of that evolution. I will deal with these chemicals later on in another chapter.

Let me take time to digress for a moment so I can explain how God has designed our ecosystem, especially as it relates to farming. First of all God designed the earth in perfect balance at its' inception. Sin has upset the balance of nature, which God is the orchestrator of. God causes to grow the right plants for the right location at the right time. Those plants provide food, shelter and habitats for other animals from microscopic organism and insects to even larger predators. Everything is perfectly coordinated even down to the bees and birds, which pollinate the plants in there search for food. If the right crop is planted that is suited for the locale, taking into consideration the climate, growing season, elevation, access to water, etc., that plant will then play host to the animal life in that area. If poisons are introduced, they not only hurt the crop, which will ultimately end up on our tables, but also the bees, birds, soil, water supply, etc. I think you get the point. The bee population in this country has been so affected by poisons that many plants are not being fertilized. It is believed that the poisons are causing the bees to not be able to direct the colony to flowers, therefore the colonies are dying. How important are bees? well every third bite of food you take is possible because of the bee. Everything is being adversely affected by greed, including us!!..Now if you still wonder why we get sicker and sicker as more and more money goes for health research, just read on. The sicker the crops become, because of the toxic poisons, the more poisons are added, the cycle continues and the end result is that the food quality has been so damaged that the nutrients have been minimized and completely destroyed and whats worst we have introduced those foreign chemicals into our bodies. When the body gets hold of a foreign substance that it cannot metabolize, that substance remains in the body because the body does not know what to do with it. That foreign substance will undoubtedly end up causing some form of cancer, unless it is removed from the system. Unless you are eating organic foods or growing your own in your backyard, you are ingesting countless chemicals daily into your body. Do you still wonder why people are dying all around us including those in the Body of Christ at an alarming rate. I just mentioned this one incident of chemical fertilization and how it started, but there are many different chemical fertilizers on the market. The bottom line is the almighty dollar. The Bible said that the love of money was the root of ALL evil. I Tim. 6:10. These corporations could care less about our health, so we have to care about our own health. It is definitely a "buyer beware" market today. The government is not protecting us because the politicians and governmental officials are being paid to pass legislation that compromises our health. You might ask who is paying them? The Lobbyist from the major corporations and the Special Interest Groups (SIG) are lining the pockets of our politicians, bureaucrats and officials, not to mention the amount of extra tax money that is generated. We as members of Christ' Body should not be surprised because Jesus said that satan is the god of this world system. Are you allowing him to take you out?

There is another demonic attack at work here to take us out and it operates through major pharmaceutical companies who are contaminating our bodies by genetically altering our foods, by tampering with seeds and seed production and producing drugs. In order to control the food market in this country these companies are altering the seeds in order to patent them for their own monetary gains. You control the seeds when you own the patent on that seed and you thereby control the food production cycle. The farmers are forced to buy these seeds or go out of business. Does this sound like a precursor to 666 or not? Not only are they getting rich off of the food production, they are the same companies who are supplying the hospitals and doctors with drugs to further contaminate you after you consume the genetically altered food products. All drugs have side effects because they have foreign substances in them that the body doesn't know what to do with, as I stated earlier. Are you still wondering why you are sick? Look at our children, who are raised on fast foods. Do you wonder why there is a rise in juvenile cholesterol levels and juvenile diabetes or why 1 in 3 kids had developed type II diabetes as of the year 2000. No telling what the rate may be today. Have you ever wondered why our youth are so angry? If the only nutrients you consume daily came from candy, potato chips and honey buns, you would be angry, violent and sick also. It was reported in 2008 that 90% of the food stamps in Detroit, Michigan were being used at liquor stores, party stores, gas stations, dollar stores, and the like. It was also reported that this same city consumed more potato chips than any other city in America. None of these outlets provided quality fresh fruits and vegetables, yet these are the stores the poor blacks are forced to shop at because there are no supermarkets in their areas. People wonder why crime is so bad in the inner cities? How can anyone think clearly eating like that, when your brain functions from the nutrients you feed it. These statistics were reported from just one major city. Think of the ramification of these facts when multiplied 1000 times across America. The up coming chapter on the link between mental health and disease will provide more information on this problem. By the way the Rockefellers' own the top 19 pharmaceutical companies in the world. I thought that I would add that interesting fact.

You might ask, why don't the farmers just grow quality food, since they own the farms?The answer to that question is, the farmers have no choice if they want to feed their families. Many farmers have actually lost their farms by not complying with the major food conglomerates, which control all aspects of mega farming. Either use their genetically modified seeds or starve to death. Most of the seed companies have been bought by these pharmaceutical giants. If you can get some seeds, you should stock up because soon you will not be able to even have a small garden in your own yard. This seems to be what is on the horizon but God will always make a way for His children. There are many companies selling seed survival kits, with good organic seeds for you to grow in an emergency or when seeds can no longer be found. People this is serious business and the long term affect will be unbelievable. I will repeat here, not all hybrid seeds are genetically modified but you should look for good quality seeds while you can and take control of your own health and the health of your family by growing a small garden! In the next chapter we will discuss in more detail what is really happening in the food industry and what if anything the government is doing to safeguard our health. I hope this information is enlightening and serves to at least give you some insight, so you can formulate a personal plan to help yourself and your family members. God has always had rams in the bushes. You can do a lot for yourself, but first you need to be informed about what is happening, then you can take charge of your own life, make some quality decisions and not leave your life in the hands of someone who serves a different god. I hate to say it, but many people are lazy, many don't exercise much discipline and still other people are just too tired and wore out to do anything about making changes. Many have no energy left when they get home from work or school, they can only pass out. They have no energy because they are living on the SAD of junk foods, drugs, chemicals, toxins and poisons!! We are more than conquerors, the Greater One lives inside of us, we can do all things through Christ who strengthens us, no weapon formed against us can prosper!! Once you make some changes you will be amazed at how you will feel. At the end of this book, I will tell you what you can do to feel great, lose weight, look younger and take a bite out of life. I will tell you what we did and if you want to, you too can feel better fast and rid yourselves of disease, sickness and pain. I don't know about you? but I am tired of family members dying of chronic diseases. My wife and I have tried counseling many of them but they refused to make changes. Wouldn't you like to be raptured out of here and not see death as a result of some chronic disease?

Key points outlined in chapter

(1)

(2)

(3)

(4)

(5)

Changes I can make to improve my health

(1)

(2)

(3)

(4)

(5)

CHAPTER THREE
LOBBYIST & GOVERNMENT AGENCIES

HOW DID LOBBYIST BECOME SO INFLUENTIAL

First of all we need to define the word lobby. I am not talking about the foyer of a building or hotel. To lobby means to influence someone to change their mind, decision or action. Therefore a lobbyist is a person who lobbies. Lobbyist have always been present to influence public policies, politicians, government agencies, etc., from the inception of our nation. In the past say fifty to sixty years or so the lobbyist have increasingly become more aggressive in their pursuits to change peoples minds, opinions, votes and actions. Many corporations and corporate giants use this method to change policies to further their financial gains or improve their bottom lines. Because many of these companies are financially able, they can be very persuasive, even to the point of bribery. Since satans' system is based on greed and the acquisition of power and mammon, many of the decision making people, including elected officials are persuaded by bribery to stand for anything, say anything and do anything. As a result of their decisions many consumers are adversely affected just because some people have no morals, are greedy for gain or exercise poor judgment. Many politicians and government officials daily vote against their conscience, deliberately are absent on crucial vote days and or blatantly lie to fatten their wallets. We as believers in the Body of Christ, should be aware of these things and govern our lives accordingly. We keep forgetting that we have an enemy who kills, steals and destroys. Don't allow yourself to get so complacent until you believe every lie of the enemy. Who's report do you believe? God's Word is His report.

These lobbyist are influencing our lives daily in many ways. These are just a few examples of how they have interfered in policy making ; by telling the FDA that a drug is safe, when it has been proven in the manufacturers' own laboratories to be harmful and this happens often. They have convinced the USDA to allow dead and diseased animals and the feces of those animals to be ground up a put in the same species food for consumption. They have influenced the USDA to allow cement to be added to animal feed to maximize the market weight of the animals. These lobbyist have been instrumental in tons of poisons being added to our food ingredients. They are responsible for 1000s' of harmful drugs flooding the market with more side effects than can be imagined. They are responsible for millions of ground up aborted fetuses being added to cosmetic products. They have influenced the FDA to approve prescription drugs that have never been properly tested. I could go on and on but I think you get the picture! One pharmaceutical laboratory had over two hundred drug recalls, which obviously meant that they were not properly testing before submitting the drugs to the FDA for approval. By the way, there are hundreds of such laboratories with recalls weekly. I only wonder what the total number of recalls have been, only God knows. Vaccinations have been approved for children, when studies had shown they cause birth defects, but lobbyist were able to influence their approval. Many of the same doctors that tell their patients to have their children vaccinated are not allowing their own children to get the same vaccinations! Why not, do they know something that they are not telling their patients? Fluoride, MSG, mercury, aspartame are all linked to health issues, yet the USDA and the FDA have been reluctant to make quality decisions to guard our health, concerning these chemicals. I will deal with the big four (fluoride, MSG, mercury and aspartame) in detail in a later chapter. Many negative decisions have been made by those in authority, which were influenced by lobbyist, that have caused countless people to suffer illnesses and even death in too many instances. I think you are finally beginning to understand that God was not kidding when he said that "the devil kills, steals and destroys", and that "the devil is the prince of this worlds' system." You may ask, how could this all be true? If this were general public knowledge, could you just imagine the number of law suits? Our judicial system would not be able to handle it. Everything I have said and will say is available public information. Satan is not concerned however with what I said, since the Church has allowed him to become this controlling. We as members in the Body of Christ should not be overly concerned either because we win, but we need to at least be aware of the enemies fiery darts. We should at least do what we can to safeguard our loved ones. We owe that much to our children.

I've said this before and before the end of this book, I will say it again. I am not downing our system of government, I am not downing any agency of our government nor am I downing any corporation, which is why I chose not to name any names. I am only reporting the truth because daily my wife and I talk to people who say, I wonder why I feel so bad, or I wonder why I can't sleep, or I have no energy or I just found out I have cancer – pray for me. We need to wake up and stop listening to our so-called experts and ask God. When God gives you the answer, be a doer of the word that He gives you. Make some changes! God is giving you many answers in this book. When you complete it, will you do business as usual or will you make some changes. Personally I am not even appalled at what is occurring in this country and the world because we the Saints have allowed things to get this bad. Satan is satan and his system is what it is, so why get upset with the devil for being the devil. We in the Body of Christ are in this world, but we do not have to be of the world. In Gods' kingdom, business is done differently. We need to enter this kingdom and do the Word as God said and show the world how heaven is. Remember our mandate to bring heaven to earth!! If you are wondering what can be done or how can I make some changes, I will give you clear, easy and rewarding suggestions at the end of this publication, just keep reading so you can be fully persuaded that change is necessary.

GOVERNMENT AGENCIES AND IMPORTANT ASSOCIATIONS
I previously mentioned some of these agencies of the government, but I will at this time explain their intended functions so we can ascertain whether they are performing their intended duties. The USDA, which stands for United States Department of Agriculture was established in 1862 by President Abraham Lin-

coln. It was established to govern food production and distribution, the quality of foods and the safeguards and concerns of the consumer through implementation of laws and regulations. It was initially established with the utmost intentions of sincerity and has served us well, but like most bureaucracies it has grown so big that it has its' flaws. Some of the leaders have allowed themselves to be bribed by lobbyist to compromise their stands on issues of concern that have been detrimental to our health and well being. This has occurred to often during the past half century in particular. The love of money being the root of all evil, is again evident.

The FDA (Food & Drug Administration) is another powerful organization within our Federal Government to assist the citizenry. It was established in 1906 and it is an agency of the United States Department of Health and Human Services. This agency is concerned with public health regulations, providing supervision of Tobacco products, dietary supplements, drugs, vaccines, bio pharmaceuticals, blood transfusions, medical devices, electromagnetic radiation, veterinary products and cosmetics.

This agency is responsible for all the synthetic drugs that are on the market. There are thousands and thousands of drugs on the market at this time and all of them had to get approved by this agency before they were released for public consumption. The real problem is the fact that every single one of these drugs have more side effects than the supposed condition (or effect) they are prescribed to treat. The main reason for such an influx in the number of drugs is of course money. It has been estimated that drug companies or pharmaceuticals annually make hundreds of billions of dollars and a few law suits here and there are not going to affect their bottom line too much. These companies and there are hundreds of them, could not generate such profits if there wasn't a demand for the drugs by the public. People knowingly and unknowingly are violating dietary laws which are leading to all sorts of illnesses and diseases and as a result they are looking for relief at any cost. Drugs really provide the license to violate the natural dietary laws instituted by God, however people don't want the consequences. The consequences are destroying our lives, causing health care to be unaffordable, costing billions in unnecessary research and polluting the environment. Our children will inherit a catastrophe, unless Jesus returns. I will mention this agency again later.

The next two agencies that will be mentioned in this book will be addressed together. These two agencies are operated in similar fashions. They are private agencies and not governmental, although they work closely with our government. They are the AMA (American Medical Association) and the ADA (American Dental Association). They are responsible for overseeing doctors and dentist. More specifically they are involved in the educational curriculum, requirements, rules and regulations, policies and licensing for all doctors and dentist and the related occupational fields. When it comes to health care in this country, these agencies are paramount and they rule with iron fist. Both doctors and dentist are virtually powerless to voice their private opinions about health care practices, procedures, etc., unless their views are in line with these agencies' views, they will suffer the consequences, which usually mean suspended or revoked licenses. Dentist and especially doctors spend too many years and too much money on their education to throw it all away for making controversial statements or giving controversial opinions. Therefore, many will remain silent even in life threatening situations at times. Their livelihood is at state. They must adhere to the policies, practices and procedures outlined by these agencies or they will suffer the consequences.

Key points outlined in chapter

(1)

(2)

(3)

(4)

(5)

Changes I can make to improve my health

(1)

(2)

(3)

(4)

(5)

CHAPTER FOUR
SICKNESS AND DISEASE IN AMERICA

PHYSICAL CAUSES OF DISEASE

This may be the most important chapter in the book! You really do need to know why you are so sick! Disease, both physical and psychological is a direct result of accumulated waste in the system that has not been eliminated and corresponding nutritional deficiencies. The accumulation of waste is referred to as "Autointoxication", which is similar to a plumbing system that is backed up so that waste can not travel through to exit. The natural body will attempt to eliminate these poisons from the system from child birth to death. These poisons are a combination of gases from undigested food, food additives, fecal matter, phlegm (mucus), antibiotics and toxins that have been deposited from poor nutritional habits, ingestion of drugs (over the counter and prescription), recreational drugs and dead foods or devitalized foods from processing. Dead foods are meats, no matter how fresh, because once the animal is killed it begins to decompose or decay. The body is literally drowning in a sea of toxic waste. When we eat devitalized, dead processed foods, it creates a sticky glue like substance that adheres to the walls of the colon. Over a period of years this build up causes the diameter of the colon to shrink so that normal bowel movement is compromised to the extent that fecal matter can't exit the system in a normal fashion. It is much like trying to run water through a stopped up water hose. The average person would be amazed at what they have lodged in their intestines. The entire length of the two intestines combined is 42 feet, which is a substantial distance for food to travel and then exit the system. They have done autopsies on people with food over two years old , still lodged in their intestines. It has been reported that bodies have actually exploded on the autopsy table during examination because of the excessive combinations of lethal toxins. Cremation chambers, used for the cremation process have actually exploded during the cremation process because of lethal concoctions of toxins in some of the corpses. Many of these toxins don't just exit the body through the normal excretion processes, because they are considered by the body to be foreign objects that the body can't identify and process properly. The gasses given off by these toxins further damage the already compromised health condition in the body. Meats take approximately four times longer to exit the body than fresh fruits and vegetables and that is under optimum conditions. When a system has been damaged over a period of years, much of the digested and undigested flesh and other waste gets trapped in the system. It was reported by the British Royal Society of Medicine that 36 known poisons have been created by this pollution process alone. Do you wonder why an alarming number of people are dying from cancers? This is just the tip of the iceberg. We will soon see an epidemic of disease and death that will be unprecedented in our history as a country. Daily drugs are being manufactured and released on the unsuspecting public at an unbelievable rate. As I mentioned earlier all drugs have side effects and the list of side effects of some drugs is unbelievable. Believe it or not the USDA and the FDA do not test drugs before they are approved for human consumption. You heard me right, they are not in the business of testing drugs. They rely on the test results from research done by the same companies that develop and market those drugs. I wonder whether their data could be flawed? These drug companies are suppose to report all known side effects, but many times the major side effects are not reported or they somehow get over looked until a few deaths have occurred. I mentioned in a previous chapter that just one pharmaceutical company, which is not considered one of the top ten, had over 200 recalls alone. All of this information may be overwhelming to you, but God has a way out for you, if you will be willing and obedient.

Food additives are another way of overloading our bodies with toxins. Virtually every packaged or process food has some additives in them. Food additives are introduced to either improve the appearance of the food, improve the taste of the food or increase the shelf life. This is the very reason why we should consume as many fruits, vegetable, legumes and grains as possible. All of the these foods are still alive and they don't need any preservation. If you don't believe that your beans, rice, wheat, split peas, etc., are still alive, just try sprouting them in a jar and see what happens. For those of you who don't know how to sprout your food items, I will give you a quick lesson at the end of the book. Sprouting is the best way to get all of the nutrients out of your food items because sprouts are alive!

Food dyes are another form of chemical that is added to foods to improve the appearance. Although finally outlawed in this country after almost 70 years of use, Red dye no. 2, was finally banned after causing numerous, birth defects, genetic damage, fetal deaths, toxicity and cancers. It has been reported that some 1 million tons of the stuff was fed to the American public before it was banned. The dyes used today are reported to be much safer. I wonder?

Uric acid which comes from the urine of animals is transmitted through the bloodstream of the animal to humans when they eat meat. This uric acid then deposits itself in the human joints which results in bone-joint dysfunctions such as arthritis, rheumatism and gout. These conditions are crippling many of our senior citizens and alarmingly even the young. The high protein an phosphorus content of meats actually leeches calcium from bones and teeth causing stooping, many fractures in the elderly and dental problems. These leeched pieces of calcium further accumulate at joints forming calcium deposits deforming the appendages and causing pain and restrictive usage. These conditions are all associated with a high meat diet.

Lets shift gears now and focus our attention on some of the pollutants that are transmitted in our water systems. Most people in this country are aware of our polluted water because the taste bears out this fact. Our drinking water has been contaminated by many companies that have dumped their toxic waste into waterways during the course of business operation. Supposedly in an effort to combat this problem the US government approved the addition of chlorine to water to kill contaminating parasites, bacteria, algae, yeast and mold. Now chlorine has it's own problems, for when it combines with natural organic matter like decaying vegetable matter it produces trihalomethames, which hardens the arteries and cause heart attacks, strokes and senility.

I mentioned earlier that I would address the fluoride situation later, so we might as well look at our fluoride problem now since we are talking about water. As I mentioned earlier, fluoride became widely available at the end of World War II, when great surpluses of the chemical was left over from the development of the atomic bomb. You heard me right! The chemical, although dangerous, was suggested as an additive to our water supply by Dr. Harold Hodge, who had worked for the Atomic Energy Commission. Dr. Hodge had been previously involved in The Manhattan Project, which deliberately gave high doses of both plutonium and radium to citizens to document their reactions in a laboratory setting. Due to his testimony and expertise, he convinced our government to add the chemical to our water supply to prevent tooth decay. Fluoridation is responsible for more than 25,000 cancer deaths per year in this country. This chemical poses risk to the brain, thyroid gland, bones and affects kidney function. Fluoride is still being used in not only water but toothpaste and other products. This has been occurring in this country for the past 60 plus years and it's use has actually been increased. Do the math 25,000 times 60 years is over 1.5 million cancer deaths associated with fluoride and counting.

Mercury is a known killer by most Americans, but did you know that one of the main ingredients in tooth fillings is mercury Do you have any fillings in your teeth? This is one of the most deadly poisons known to man, yet daily people are getting dental fillings with mercury being 50% of the filling ingredients. Just because your fillings may be old, don't think that the danger has passed. The toxic gas vapors from mercury have been documented escaping from fillings over fifty years old! You heard me right, fillings fifty years old are still affecting your health today. Only God knows how much damage has been done in our bodies. Some of the dangers associated with mercury are outlined. Minute particles of mercury can cause symptoms ranging from feeling listless, fatigued, depressed, irritable and if swallowed, sever poisoning and even death. Many Americans have had those old fillings removed, but many more are not aware that they are posing any health threat to them. The ADA has not allowed dentist to reveal to their patients the risk that are involved. The dentist and dental assistants as well as the patients are all exposed to this problem. Mercury poisoning is highly toxic and is a silent threat.

Many Americans love to ingest some of the sugar substitutes that are on the market in an effort to reduce their sugar intake. Beware of the substitute you take and read your labels. Aspartame, being one, is highly dangerous to infants and can freely pass the placental barrier causing physical and mental birth defects. We in the Body of Christ need to at least be aware of this situation because aspartame is being used as a substitute because it is sixteen times sweeter than sugar. Aspartame has a list of side effects that are too numerous to mention, 92 to be exact, including the ultimate side effect, death. Is it still on the market? Of course it is on the market and being used in more and more products daily. At this writing it is in over 40 products. It is extremely profitable so it may take many more deaths before it is removed from the consumer market. Change comes slowly when profits are involved, irregardless of the severity! Google aspartame for yourself and do your own investigation. It is in many of the diet products on the market, so chances are you have some aspartame in your house at this moment. Many diabetics are ingesting this substitute, however it has been reported that it further worsens existing diseases like diabetes by causing complications. If you are a diabetic, did you know that? There are some safer sugar substitutes that have been used for years. Later I will share some of these with you.

Although there are many other harmful chemicals on the market that you should be cognizant of, I can't name them all. This book would be too long and you would be bored. However I saved the best or I should say the most interesting chemical for last.

The last chemical that I will mention is MSG. This one is interesting because it causes you to want to eat more and more and more. Have you wondered why we have such an obesity problem now and especially with our young people? MSG (monosodium glutamate) is a chemical that is used to flavor foods. It first was introduced on a large scale in this country by the Chinese, who included it in virtually all their dishes. America is in love with Chinese food. As a matter of fact Chinese food is the most widely eaten food in America besides American food. There are more Chinese restaurants in America than any other restaurant. I must admit that I am partial to Chinese food myself, but when I do eat it, especially at a restaurant, I will ask them if they cook with MSG. If they say that they do, my wife and I will exit gracefully, no matter how good their food is. Monosodium glutamate is another toxic food additive. Have you ever noticed that you just can't get enough of Chinese food and that when you finish within an hour or so you can eat more? That reason is linked to MSG, which they use generously in practically all their dishes. This is the kicker, MSG has a substance in it that tells the brain that it needs more. In other words it shuts off the "stop mechanism" in your brain, which tells your body that you are full. There is one more food item that everyone consumes daily that does the same thing. Keep reading I will reveal that product to you later! I will come back to this important point. MSG is linked to a disease called "Kwok" or another name for it is "Chinese Restaurant Syndrome". The symptoms of this disorder are characterized by numbness, burning sensations, tingling, facial pressure & tightness, chest pains, headaches, nausea, rapid heart beat, drowsiness, weakness and difficult breathing for asthmatics. These side effects don't occur in all people, so this particular drug will be on the market for decades. You just need to be aware of it's symptoms so you can monitor your own health. Annually 1.1 million tons of MSG is consumed world wide. It is obviously a money maker. What MSG does is it blends with and rounds off the total perception of other tastes. MSG by itself is nasty, but when it combines with natural food flavors, it tends to enhance them. MSG has been around for years and despite public pressure it is still being used. It is in virtually all of the packaged processed foods and is marketed under different names. It is present in many seasoning and in flavor enhancers. The most important point that I wanted to mention is the fact that when it was discovered that MSG turns off the brain's "you are full switch", food producers were thrilled because that meant that you would consume more and more of their products. MSG is in all fast foods, chips, snacks, etc,. These are foods that our children love, yet we wonder why they are so obese as well as many adults, also who eat unhealthy diets because they are hungry but pressed for time! We need to stop being lazy and be more proactive in the

preparation of our own family meals. If you are concerned about MSG and its' effects, be aware of the following product names because they all have the same reactive components:
Autolyzed Plant Protein
Sodium Caseinate
Calcium Caseinate
Textured Protein
Yeast Extract
Yeast Food
Yeast Nutrient
Autolyzed Yeast
Natural Flavors

LEARN TO READ YOUR LABELS AND IF YOU CAN'T PRONOUNCE IT, LEAVE IT!

Key points outlined in chapter

(1)

(2)

(3)

(4)

(5)

Changes I can make to improve my health

(1)

(2)

(3)

(4)

(5)

CHAPTER FIVE
TODAYS HEALTH CARE DILEMMA

HEALTH CARE INDUSTRY STATISTICS

We are going to review some statistics at this time, so please bear with me because this is vital for you to see where we are and where we are headed. I believe that if you see these facts, they will prompt you to at least make an effort to become more health conscious as you chose what you consume, for these statistics will show you what we as a nation are facing concerning healthcare cost now and in the immediate future.

Most health care facilities are privately owned but the government is responsible for 60 – 65% of the health care insurance in this country. This insurance is paid through the Medicare, Medicaid, Tricare and Childrens' Health Care programs. In the United States 49.9 million Americans are uninsured. The United States pays twice as much for health care expenditures, yet lags behind all the other wealthy nations. Our infant mortality and life expectancy rates for infants are astounding. Our life expectancy rate is ranked at 42nd in the world and our life expectancy rate at birth ranks at 50th among leading nations. These are statistics furnished by the World Health Organization (WHO). The alarming thing is, we rank 1st in healthcare cost of expenditure, yet 37th in performance and even worst, only 72nd in level of care. That just should not be. How can we be spending so much, yet getting so little? In 2006 the United States accounted for 75% of the world's biotechnology revenues and 82% of the world's research and development in biotechnology. What type of returns are we receiving for such capital outlays? For those that don't know, biotechnology is the field of applied biology that involves the use of living organisms and bioprocesses in engineering, technology and medicine. Biotechnology is concerned with genetic engineering, cell and tissue culture technology and breeding programs that include artificial selection and hybridization. Currently the United States is spending 20% of it's GDP (Gross Domestic Product) revenue on health care. The following figures will explain in dollars and cents how this all impacts the American people as individuals.

AVERAGE FAMILY OF 4 HEALTH INSURANCE PRE-MIUM SINCE THE YEAR 2000

YEAR	INDIVIDUAL	FAMILY
2000	$2471	$6438
2001	$2689	$7061
2002	$3083	$8003
2003	$3383	$9068
2004	$3695	$9950
2005	$4024	$10880
2006	$4242	$11480
2007	$4479	$12106

2008 $4704 $12680
2009 $4824 $13375

At the end of this year 2012, it has been projected that the average cost for health insurance for the family of four will be an incredible $20, 000 yearly!!! Nobody but the rich could afford that. This is why President Obama is trying hard to push his health care proposal, which I personally oppose and I will tell you why. Why should I pay for your healthcare, when you choose to violate God's dietary laws, which in turn leads to your illness? I choose to obey God and He is my insurer! I personally am against abortion also and part of this mandatory health program will fund abortions! The above figures clearly indicate that we are in trouble concerning our healthcare expenditures and it will only get worst as we daily discover new drugs, which will only serve to license continual poor nutritional choices and lead to more costly side effects.

WHY OUR HEALTH CARE SYSTEM HAS FAILED

Now that you understand what we as a nation are up against and you have a better understanding of our current health care system, let's now see how it got so bad. From the Word of God, the Holy Bible, we in the Body of Christ know that God said that this world system would fail. The reason it will fail is because it was designed and is being run by satan and his children. Satan cannot design anything that will run with perfection because he is a defeated foe who can only "kill, steal and destroy" John 10:10. When any being has an MO based on killing, stealing and destroying, failure is inevitable. John 14:30 says that satan is the (prince) god of this world. It is referring to this world's systems or methods of operation. For this very reason the financial system, educational system, judicial system and the health care systems are all failing miserably. When the foundation of your very being is not love, failure is inevitable. God is love, John 4:24. It is for this very reason that God created this world for us, because He loved us. He created a perfect world for His children with everything in perfect balance. I mentioned in an earlier chapter that sin upset the balance of this world. Sin continues to prevail. If it were not for the love of money and the greed for power, we would not have a health care dilemma. God gave us the plants to not only eat but to cure the ailments that we encounter. We in the Body of Christ can't keep letting food take us out before our time. The main reason why plants, in particular herbs, are not stressed as cures for diseases is because you cannot patent a plant and thereby profit financially from it. If you could patent a plant then many of the drugs on the market, with all their side effects, would never had been developed. Now some doctors, those whose consciences have finally condemned them, have given up their medical practices and are promoting herbs and natural methods of curing diseases. Many of these doctors are prescribing herbs for their patients and are achieving remarkable results. There are many Naturopathic doctors practicing today who believe in letting the body cure itself as God designed it. Another thing that is occurring, is the practice of adding some synthetic ingredient to a herb or plant to get a patent. Herbs work best in their natural state as God made them. The true fact is herbs do work, my immediate family and I have been using them over 40 years and my parents and grandparents before us as well.

Because we are talking about the healthcare system, we need to understand the role of the nutritionist. There are two schools of thought on the subject of nutrition. Lets talk about the nutrition your traditional nutritionist advocate. These individuals graduated from the fully accredited colleges and universities. Their courses of study were set up to agree with the world's system, which again is based on killing, stealing and destroying. They are taught to agree with the FDA, USDA, AMA, ADA, etc., and as a result they are licensed to give the public what they have been taught. Most of what they were taught is good but a lot of it is in error. They were taught to condone the usage of drugs. They were taught that milk does a body good and is therefore required for calcium . They were taught that your basic intake of protein should come from meat. They were taught that you should eat three meals a day. They were taught that calorie intake is important and that you should count them. If you eat a diet of primarily fruits and vegetables, you don't need to count calories because these foods are low in calories. You only need to be concerned with calorie counting if you are eating the SAD of poor nutritional foods. Basically these nutritionist mimic the authoritarian mandates of the above associations and agencies and are discouraged from voicing any opinions to the contrary, because their licensing is controlled by the AMA.

The next group of nutritionist, of which I am one, are Holistic Nutritionist and we approach nutrition from the foundational premise that man is a tripartite being. In I Thess. 5:23 the Bible mentions that we have a tripartite nature. We are spirits, we live in bodies and we possess souls. When you minister to an individual from that point of view, you will treat the person much differently. This approach to nutrition is based on the biblical concept of health and wholeness and functions to assist the body in it's attempt to heal itself. We further are opposed to the ingestion of drugs because they are synthetic and thereby the cause of further problems, which result from their side effects. We also are opposed to drugs because they further poison the body with harmful toxins. We suggest the eating of foods that are alive and not dead because dead foods have begun the decomposing and decaying process. Since you are feeding a live body, the body should be feed live food for optimum health and longevity. We also know that to violate these practices only opens the door for disease to attack and destroy the body. We also realize that it is possible to get all the necessary nutrients you need from fruits, vegetables, nuts and grains. We further realize that plants (herbs) can be used to alleviate illnesses and that God has caused to grow everything you need to sustain you in this world. We also teach that good health will return to those who rid themselves of all toxins and then strengthen the body with the proper foods. It was Hippocrates who said "food should be for your medicine and medicine for your food". In case you didn't know, he was the father of modern medicine. It is his distinguished oath that doctors swear to before they can be licensed - "The Hippocratic Oath". He was quoting the Bible, when he made that statement. Ezel. 47:12, Rev. 22:2. I know Hippocrates would probably decline to practice medicine today, since it relies so much on drugs. He lived 400 years before Christ and apparently agreed with God, as his statement bears out. Just like this country was founded on Godly principles, and we have transgressed them, so was modern medicine. We have accomplished so much in modern medicine, yet we have regressed in some of the more basic elementary practices. Before I end this chapter, I would like to say again that I personally am not attacking anybody, their profession or even their ideals. I am addressing the Body of Christ and expect that we will do better because we are accountable for what we know. Luke 12:48. God said that He would not have us ignorant concerning the wiles of the devil. Eph. 6:11. God also said that we should know the truth and the truth we know shall set you free.

John 8:32. So far I have endeavored to bring you truths, please respond accordingly.

PRESCRIPTION DRUG COST

The cost for prescription drugs are also a major dilemma. Many patients are on multiple prescriptions, as many as fifteen or more in some cases. Although they may have medical insurance to cover the major portion of the cost, many patients are still stressed by the cost of the co-pay. We had a close family member, now deceased, who died in her fifties from cancer. Prior to her death, she had complained about the cost of one of her many prescribed drugs. I can't remember the name of the drug but she complained that each pill cost her $100.00. Mind you this was just for one of her many prescribed medicines. We agreed with her that the amount seemed ridiculous but that is what she had to pay. Obviously the medication didn't save her! I have since gone online to do some research on prescription drug cost and I was amazed to find out the retail cost verses the actual manufactured cost. We all know that any company in the United States that does business is doing it for a profit. That is a given but the markup on some products is unbelievable Below is a simple chart outlining some of the information I discovered on some popular drugs.

RETAIL DRUG COST	MANUFACTURES COST
100 Zoloft 50mg = $206.80	$1.75 per tablet/capsule
100 Claritin 10mg = $215.17	$0.71 per tablet/capsule
100 Prilosec 20mg = $360.97	$0.52 per tablet/capsule
100 Prozac 20mg = $247.47	$0.11 per tablet/capsule
100 Xanax 1mg = $136.79	$0.02 per tablet/capsule

For some of the rarer diseases, the cost for drugs would astound you. For example the drug called SOLIRIS cost $409,500 per year or $1122.00 per day.

The drug ELAPRASE cost $375,000 per year or $1027.00 per day.

Mind you these drugs are for rare diseases but from the above information, I believe you can see how profitable drugs have become, or I should say, see how profitable we have allowed them to become. The cost to develop some of these drugs is also astounding. For instance it was reported that 800 million was invested in the R&D of the above mentioned drug Soliris. When a company invests that much in a product, what is the likelihood of it not being approved, nor ever recalled regardless of the side effects? You tell me.

Key points outlined in chapter

(1)

(2)

(3)

(4)

(5)

Changes I can make to improve my health

(1)

(2)

(3)

(4)

(5)

CHAPTER SIX
MAJOR DISEASES AND THEIR SYMPTOMS

CARDIOVASCULAR DISEASE OR HEART DISEASE

Cardiovascular disease is the most prevalent major disease in America today, killing more than 459,000 people annually. Cardiovascular disease, which I will just call heart disease from now on, is a class of diseases that involve the heart or blood vessels (arteries and veins). While the term technically refers to any disease that affects the cardiovascular system, it is often used to refer to those related to arteriosclerosis and or hypertension. The causes, mechanisms and treatments of these conditions often overlap. Cardiovascular deaths and diseases have increased at an astonishingly fast rate in low and middle class individuals, due most often to poor nutritional choices. These poor choices are primarily made based on ignorance, however increasingly the bad choices stem from the lack of good quality food availability in poorer areas.

Although heart disease usually affects older adults, it is increasingly being detected in younger adults and even in children. This is obviously caused by the poor diets of many of our young people, which we will discuss later. The antecedent or precursor of heart disease, notably arteriosclerosis begins in early life, making primary prevention efforts necessary from childhood. There are two primary factors that lead to heart disease. One is high levels of bad cholesterol and the other is hypertension or high blood pressure. Both of these conditions will lead directly to heart disease if not addressed as soon as detected.

Cholesterol is the organic chemical substance classified as a waxy steroid of fat. It is an essential structural component in cell membranes. Cholesterol is required to establish proper cell membrane permeability and fluidity. Now that we know what it is and the fact that it is required to sustain a healthy body, let's see why it can lead to heart disease. Bad cholesterol is the culprit and it is manufactured in the body as a by product of harmful foods. Fats from saturated oils, trans fats, red meat, butter, cheese, ice cream and processed foods made with trans fats from partially hydrogenated oils all lead to bad cholesterol. These cholesterol deposits, which are like sticky glue, adhere to the walls of the arteries and travel throughout the circulatory system wreaking havoc. Before I go on, I want to explain what hydrogenated oils are and why they are so harmful to the body and lead to bad cholesterol.

Hydrogenated oils are oils that have had hydrogen gas forced into them to mimic the taste of butter and it is used in the following products. Crackers, cookies, frozen waffles, pudding, peanut butter, cereal bars, prepared frozen foods, most prepared foods, soup (canned and powered), salad dressings and many more food items contain this deadly oil. Watch your ingredient list. This type of oil has been directly linked to heart disease, cancer, diabetes, multiple sclerosis and only time will tell what other maladies. There are good oils on the market that your body can utilize like olive or safflower and oils from nuts and fish. The human body can't properly metabolize the hydrogen gas and the separating of the oil by the gas causes the body to reject the oil.

Hypertension is better known as high blood pressure and many African Americans suffer with this condition. It is directly linked to poor nutritional habits. The blood pressure becomes high when the bloodstream is impure due to waste, poisons, fat deposits and toxins. God said in His Word that the life of the flesh is in its' blood. Lev. 17:11. When the bloodstream is full of impurities, the heart has to overwork to pump the blood through the system, thereby increasing the pressure. The fact that so much waste is in the blood and that the heart has to over-work, creates conditions for the heart to stop, or for an individual to have either a stroke, where clogged veins in the brain are involved or a heart attack, where clogged arteries or heart valves are involved. It all boils down to the SAD of nutritionally poor foods and drugs which help to poison the system. Eliminate the poisons and toxins, eat a predominantly organic plant based diet and watch your health issues disappear. As far as the consumption of fat goes, God directs us to not eat it. Lev. 7:23

THE NEXT MAJOR DISEASE IS DIABETES

Diabetes (formerly called Sugar Diabetes), until the sugar industry coerced the AMA to drop the word sugar from the disease, is primarily a disease characterized by the body's inability
to produce natural insulin. Insulin, which is a natural hormone
is produced and normally secreted by the pancreas into the
bloodstream and it regulates and converts sugars into energy.
Due to a poor diet of processed foods, sugars (the number one
drug in the world and one of the most addictive), fats and drugs
or toxins, the pancreas becomes clogged by mucous so that it
cannot secrete insulin. As a result any sugar consumed will be
converted into fats instead of energy, due to the insulin deficiency and diabetics become obese. By the way obesity is almost synonymous with diabetes. When a person is diagnosed
with diabetes, he or she is prescribed artificial insulin which is
made of drugs (toxins) or pig insulin. The insulin, either type,
whether in pills or injected make the circulation problems
caused by the sugars being converted to fats rather than energy,
even worst. Due to poor circulation, doctors elect to amputate
the patients limbs. All of this could be avoided if the system
were just flushed of all poisons and toxins. Once the amputation
process starts, doctors will continue to cut until there isn't much
of the patient left. It is all about the MONEY. If you were
healed, you would not be paying the salary of the professionals.
Another problem associated with this condition is that the patients are told to continue to eat sugar to supposedly control
their insulin..This continued consumption of sugar and the artificial insulin further compromises the blood which is normally
filtered through the kidneys. The kidneys will ultimately fail
and the patient is told he or she will need a kidney transplant or
kidney dialysis treatments. Kidney dialysis is the process of
cleaning the blood and recirculating it back into system. The

problem is that the cleaning procedure uses even more drugs (toxins), How can anyone effectively clean anything with toxins, you tell me? The next occurrence in this diabetic cycle is death!! The patient could have lived a long life with all their members intact, but it would not have prospered the medical profession, who apparently care more about ones money than ones life. The amount of money made on such a patient is staggering. That downward spiraling health cycle of the diabetic that we just outlined is due to poor eating habits, trusting doctors and medical practitioners, not taking enough responsibility for ones own health and being lazy or undisciplined. Does this describe you? I hope not! One very alarming fact about this condition called diabetes is that 90% of the people who have to undergo kidney dialysis treatment, which is often required as a result of diabetes, are African-Americans. African -Americans have to really reevaluate their dietary habits and stop believing all their doctors say, as if he or she were a God.

ONE OF THE DEADLIEST KILLERS – CANCER

What is cancer in the first place and where did it come from? There are more than 100 different kinds of cancer, but 100 years ago it was virtually unknown. We will find out what occurred that caused such a killer to be unleashed on the American people, what you can do to avoid being its' next victim and the myth called cancer research. Cancer is defined by The National Cancer Institute as a disease "in which abnormal cells divide without control and are able to invade other tissues". Cancer can thus spread to other parts of the body through the blood and lymph systems.

There are five basic cancer groups:
1) Carcinoma – cancer that starts in the skin
2) Sarcoma – cancer that starts in the bone or musculo – skeletal system
3) Leukemia – cancer that starts in blood forming tissue such as bone marrow
4) Lymphoma or myeloma – cancer that starts in the lymphatic or immune systems
5) Central nervous system – cancer that starts in the brain, spinal column or nervous system

The 10 most prevalent cancers in the order of their occurrence are :
1) Non-melanoma skin cancer – associated with exposure to the sun and the elements
2) Lung – associated primarily with cigarette smoking
3) Breast – primarily involving females
4) Prostate – associated with male gland that assist in production of seminal fluid
5) Colorectal – associated with the intestines and where they terminate at the anal opening
6) Bladder- associated with urine retention and secretion
7) Melanoma – frequently from moles associated with deeper skin problems in the melanin
8) Lymphatic – associated with and involving the lymph nodes
9) Kidney – associated many times with patients with diabetes on dialysis
10) Leukemia – associated with blood

There is a dietary link to the development of cancer in the body. Although there are many different types, a healthy lifestyle characterized by a plant base diet of fresh fruits, vegetables with grains and nuts, plenty of exercise and a generally healthy environment can minimize and even prevent a person from developing this dreaded disease. Much like a plant – when a plant is healthy and wholesome, it attracts very few if any insects or pest. On the other hand an unhealthy plant attracts every parasite. Healthy organism are strong enough to ward off diseases. In the case of our human bodies, God has equipped us with a strong enough immune system to ward off all diseases, provided that we have not compromised our ability to fight off sickness and disease by our improper diets of chemicals, toxins, drugs and waste, which unfortunately often describe exactly what we are eating! Those cancerous cells that take over the body are composed of foreign matter or poisons that have been introduced to the body and in combination with other toxins wreak havoc on the entire system. Some of these poisonous substances actually attack the normal cells and cause them to change or mutate. The good news is, all of this can be reversed in the body and optimum health can return, if the body is cleansed of these poisons and then feed the proper nutritious foods. Cancer does not have to be a death sentence for people. Later I will outline some things that have been done by others who are completely cancer free at this writing. If they can take control of their lives, so can you with some information, a little discipline and a change in habits. The real problem has been that people were never told that they should walk in divine health their entire lives. I am telling you that you can. I have said this before but I believe it bears repeating. Most health care professionals really believe what they have been taught and don't think that optimum health is possible for a patient an, especially for those with chronic diseases. You can't blame a person for not knowing. Most doctors actually are convinced that the treatments and drugs that they are administering are the best remedy for your ailments. We humans want to do as we please and eat what we want, but not suffer for it. That simply is impossible. You cannot violate natural laws and not pay the consequences. Because we have determined to violate these laws, the medical professionals are devising ways for us to do just that by developing drugs for everything. The problem is someone has to pay, and you are paying with chronic health conditions and outrageous medical bills.

There has been some remarkable discoveries concerning cancer in the last twenty years. In the United States we are just hearing about the work of Dr. Tullio Simoncini, which began about twenty years ago. His discovery has revolutionized the field for those who have accepted his research. The AMA has not even acknowledged his work. He is one of the worlds' leading oncologist or cancer doctors, who resides in Italy. Even in his own country they have not accepted his findings or acknowledged the patients cured using his method. You heard me right, 99% of his patents are cured and most within days or weeks. He has lost his medical license and is facing a three year term in prison. Apparently The Italian government is just as uninterested as ours in terms of valuing human lives. Satan is the prince of this worlds' system, not just the American system. The problem with Dr. Simoncini' cure is that it is done by using sodium bicarbonate or baking soda, which can be purchased at any $0.99 store. As I mentioned earlier in this book, if no patent can be obtained on a product, nobody seems to be interested. You can not obtain a patent on sodium bicarbonate because it is a natural product. Whether it cures cancer or not, if no money can be made, a saved life is not important.

The doctor was so troubled by the death of so many people and especially children from the cancer disease that he asked the Lord what causes cancer and what will cure it. In his private prayer time the Lord told him that cancer was a fungus and just like any fungus it spreads rapidly. Dr. Simoncini was told by the Lord that simple baking soda would kill the fungus on contact. When cancers are internal the Dr. uses catheters or injections to

64

kill the cancer fungus. The fungus is known as candida albicans. If you want more information on this revolutionary finding and the treatment method, just google Dr. Tullio Simoncini. Don't even bother to ask your doctor about this because he can only respond as directed by the AMA, even if he or she wanted to suggest this treatment. People all around the world are rushing to his defense as they consider him a hero. Do your own investigation!

DISEASES CAUSED BY MINERAL DEFICIENCIES

There are other diseases caused by mineral deficiencies instead of vitamin deficiencies, which occur again because of poor nutritional choices. Whether it is a vitamin deficiency , mineral deficiency, amino acid deficiency or any deficiency, it all results from poor nutritional decisions. The following diseases occur as a result of mineral deficiencies:

Anemia	Heart Disease	Pneumonia
Acid conditions	Intestinal Diseases	Rheumatism
Appendicitis	Malnutrition	Rickets
Cancer	Menstrual disorders	Sciatica
Colitis	Nerve conditions	Scurvy
Constipation	Neuritis	Tetany
Convulsions	Pellagra	Tuberculosis
Diabetes	Paralysis	Tumors
Dysentery	Infantile paralysis	Skin eruptions
Eczema	Pleurisy	

Key points outlined in chapter

(1)

(2)

(3)

(4)

(5)

Changes I can make to improve my health

(1)

(2)

(3)

(4)

(5)

CHAPTER SEVEN
THE CLEANSING PROCESSES

It is vitally important that you periodically cleanse your bodies. This is extremely important if you live on the standard American diet (SAD) of fast foods, processed foods, packaged foods, instant foods, meats, cheeses, dairy products, eggs and or you take any drugs, whether over the counter or prescription. That just about includes everyone. The fact is our bodies are so over loaded with poisons, toxins, chemicals, waste and undigested food until it is really a testimony to God that we haven't died already! For us to live to seventy or even eighty under these conditions is remarkable and shows God's grace and mercy. I mentioned this in the beginning of this book but because it is important to the topic at hand I will reiterate now. In biblical times dietary constraints were not emphasized because their food choices were limited to what they could grow on the land, raise on the land, as far as live stock and forge for in the wild. Unlike us who have all kinds of food products available, they were extremely limited. Our complex lifestyles, ability to eat foods from around the world, advances in science and general complacency concerning dietary disciplines, puts us at risk to not only develop health problems but die from ignorance of basic laws and lack of common sense concerning what we put in our bodies. We should all live past one hundred in good health and then only die when we had completed our assignments as Moses had. The Bible says that Moses was 120 years old when he died, yet his eyesight was clear and he was as strong as ever. Deut. 34:7,8. We have been promised the same 120 years according to God's Word and when we go we should go because our God given assignments have been completed, not because some disease took us out. We have a better covenant, based on better promises than Moses did. What is our excuse? Are we letting the idol of food destroy our temples and curtail our efforts to be used by God?

NATURAL CLEANSING AND DETOXING

Detoxing and cleansing is basically the same thing, the words can be used synonymously. You should detox at least once a year. My mother would usually detox us at the beginning of each year. Many people have never detoxed, so if that is you, you definitely need to do it. The body can throw off most waste naturally through the normal excretion processes that the body uses, however due to our SAD our systems are so clogged that the normal processes of elimination have been compromised and are not functioning optimally. Just like we have a need for plumbers occasionally because our drainage or septic systems get clogged, our bodies also get clogged. When a plumber is needed, it does not mean that the systems are not working, just clogged. By the same reasoning, even if our systems of elimination are working well, we do get clogged from time to time.

When there is a clog in your elimination system it will not go away by itself. The problem needs to be addressed or it will result in a health crisis later on or even a disease which can lead to death. That neglect of an apparent problem is crucial.

Natural or normal detoxing occurs daily in our bodies through the various organs associated with the elimination of waste. In case you were not aware of your internal functions, I have outlined a simple explanation of the organs involved and how they are designed to function. Unless you took anatomy classes, you would not be too familiar with your organs and how they are suppose to function.

Waste and toxins travel through your blood to your LIVER, which filters the blood removing the impurities. Toxins and poisons are also eliminated through the KIDNEYS, which filter the liquid and then produces the urine or uric acids and impurities. This is the reason urine is yellow in color and not clear like the water you initially drink. After your food is thoroughly masticated or chewed the bulk waste goes into the upper INTESTINES then the lower INTESTINES before being eliminated through the rectum.

Waste in the form of gaseous poison or toxic vapors are filtered through the LUNGS.

The LYMPH NODES are the filtering organs for lymph fluid which is in the blood. Lymph fluid enters and exits the blood through capillaries. Lymph fluid takes nutrients, oxygen and hormones to each cell and removes toxins, poisons and waste from each cell and takes that waste to one of the 600 – 700 LYMPH NODES for filtering. Afterward the lymph fluid is recycled back into the bloodstream to begin the process over again.

The final organ of elimination is the SKIN, which is the largest organ in the body, it filters out poisons and waste and excretes them in the form of perspiration. If your body is clogged with poisons, undoubtedly your pores are clogged also to some extent. Perspiration removes much waste excreted through the skin. This is one good benefit of exercise.

CLEANSING AND DETOXING METHODS THAT WE CAN DO
Usually when you read or hear about cleansing or detoxing, it will normally be referring to the removable of waste from the colon or intestines. However removing waste from the bloodstream is just as crucial. It was God who said that "life of anything living is in the blood". Lev.17:11, 14. If the life is in the blood then the death must also be associated with the blood. Actually Naturopathic doctors will tell you that the death of a person begins in the colon and the blood. The cleansing and detoxing methods we have employed address the entire body because waste, poisons and toxins can accumulate in any area of the body. Since we are what we eat, our individual bodies are different. We don't all eat the SAD, which I defined earlier. When my wife and I detox, we don't have to employ all of these techniques because we have been health conscious for years and as a result we have gradually made changes that have improved our health. If you have never detoxed, then most of what I will outline can be incorporated into your regimen. If however you have been eating healthy organic foods and no sugars, processed foods or packaged foods and a minimal amount of meats and not taking any drugs, you may not need to detox. You have to be your own judge, because you know your

70

own body best, or you should.

There are nine things that will occur while you are doing the detoxing.

(1) You will rest your organs through fasting

(2) You will stimulate your liver to drive toxins from your body

(3) You will promote elimination through the intestines, kidneys and skin

(4) You will improve your blood circulation

(5) You will refuel your body with healthy nutrients

(6) You will eliminate undigested food

(7) You will energize yourself and regain your healing ability

(8) you will lose weight

(9) Your skin will glow and feel vibrant and clear of any bumps or blemishes.

Detoxing and cleansing will address every single cell in your body. If you are ready, I will outline what we have done and do on a regular basis. You are free to try these methods if you so desire. We and others like us have benefited tremendously from detoxing. People have actually gotten out of wheelchairs, recovered from strokes, thrown away their glasses and have experienced the gamut of health recoveries, including complete healing from cancers. It is more powerful than you could imagine. God wants you whole and in divine health. If you try this, you will be amazed at your personal results.

The best way for you to begin this process is to start juicing. I will go into more details about the juicing method in the next paragraph. For those of you who are just addicted to eating food, then you can begin by doing a colon cleanse and a liver cleanse or liver flush. There are many good products on the market that you can use for this purpose. They are sold at the health food stores. It is a way for you to begin detoxing your body. You will be amazed at the amount of garbage you have in your system. There is a very easy way to tell whether you need cleansing or not! Multiply 3 meals a day by 7 days and you get 21 meals per week. Now multiply the number of toilet visits you make daily times the 7 days, then subtract the toilet visits from the number of meals. If your tally is zero, then you wont need a colon cleanse You are suppose to go three times a day if you eat three full meals per day. When one meal enters the system, the previous meal should be exiting. This is ideal for a person in optimal health. Waste should never be allowed to stay in the system for any period of time. If you only have one toilet visit per day for 7 days, you would have 14 meals still trapped in your system. If this build up continues over a period of time, it can lead to "autointoxication" or poisoning of the system. It was determined during the autopsy of a famous actor, whose name I will not mention, that he had 75 lbs. of fecal matter lodged in his colon at his death. When you do the cleansing and discover how much better you feel, I believe you will be motivated to do a complete juice fast for at least 14 days. This fast will assist your body in rejuvenating and further cleansing.

For the juicing process to work properly, you have to be committed and not cheat because you will not gain the benefits. In order to do this properly, you should have a juicer , blender, and food processor. It does not matter what models, for any model will work. Unless you have a decent juicer however, there may be certain fruits and or vegetables that will be difficult for you to process properly. Don't let that stop you though. As you see the marvelous results, you will be glad to invest in better equipment later and you will incorporate this juicing fast into your regular dietary regimen. Use only organic fruits and vegetables, with the exception of a few produce, which are usually fit for consumption even if they may not be organic. These include pineapples, avocados, bananas, mangoes, lemons, limes, peppers and cucumbers if you definitely can't find organic ones. In the case of cucumbers, if they are not organic, then make sure you peel them. You can go online to find out other produce that don't necessarily have to be organic. The point is to use as many organic produce as you can get. It should be obvious that you don't want to put anymore chemicals or toxins in your body than you already have. It would defeat the purpose of the juice fast. Normally when a person eats, they should not mix fruits with vegetables because the body digest fruit in 15 – 20 minutes and it takes longer to digest vegetables and of course even longer to digest meats. When the fruit, vegetables and meats are eaten at one time, the body will not digest the food properly because the enzymes used to digest one food group is different than the enzymes used to digest another food group. What results is undigested food stuck in your system. In the case of juicing, that is not a problem because the nutrients are entering the body in a liquid state and are immediately assimilated into the bloodstream and utilized by the system. As far as combinations go, when you start, be creative and make juices that are pleasant to you. If you don't, you may get discouraged and give up. Have fun with it. Remember fruits are primarily for cleansing the body and vegetables are for building, repairing and maintaining the body. Make sure you still drink your 8 glasses of water or more each day to assist the body in flushing the poisons from the entire system. Your first few days will be the hardest because your body is addicted to chewing food and enjoying its' delicacies. If you can fight through the first few days, it will get easier as time goes by. Remember you are not starving your body just feeding your body nutrients, without chewing. Theoretically you could live a long time without actually chewing. Comatose patients and those on intravenous feeding programs do it all the time and many actually gain weight. I am not trying to be funny in saying that. I am merely reassuring you that you wont die in the process of juicing, regardless of the length of time you do it!

There is another side to juicing and that is the healing crisis episodes that will occur. The healing process is inevitable and unpredictable, depending on your true state of health. This occurs after your body has gotten use to the fasting process. Depending on your individual body, it may occur after only three days, but usually more like a week or so. This is indicative of the body repairing itself and it could result in rashes, sore throats, running noses, coughing up phlegm and mucous, watery eyes, itching, bumps or blemishes, etc. This is very individualistic and it depends on what damage has been done on your particular body. The body has to correct itself and it will do so, if given the right conditions. That is the beauty of the juice fast. When this occurs be joyous because you are healing! Your body gets bombarded with nutrients directly into the bloodstream, so it is not a wonder that miraculous things can and have occurred quickly. I think I should repeat something I mentioned earlier. Our bodies are looking for nutrients, not beautiful dishes, aromatic cuisines, pleasant entrees or sweeten delicacies. When you finally give the body what it has been longing for, watch out, no telling what can occur, but it will be all good. Juicing is like taking megadoses of nutrients. God has tried to prepare our meals for us. When you juice and reap the results, you will finally appreciate what God has done. So when you go through the healing process, don't give up and quit because it is necessary for you to walk in divine health. When you start feeling the discomforts, just remember your healthy breakthrough is just on the other side. Many people have been able to cease all their prescribed drugs at the end of their fast. I am not telling you to throw away your medicines, but after a doctors' check up, he will tell you whether you need your meds anymore or not. Another common occurrence after about three days, is the lost of weight. In some cases the weight can come off so fast that it shocks some people. I remember one fast I was on where I lost over 40 lbs in just 13 days. The weight lost actually caused me to discontinue the fast. I was beginning to look like a terminally ill cancer patient because I had lost so much weight in such a short amount of time. Under normal circumstances that would be too much weight to lose in such a short amount of time, but when juicing expect the weight to really come off fast!

The following fruits and vegetables are extremely beneficial during a juice fast because they really are nutritionally power-ful. All dark green leafy vegetables, avocados, blackberries, blueberries, tomatoes, mangoes, cantaloupes, watermelons, honeydew melons, bananas, butternut squash, zucchinis, sweet potatoes, beets, celery, carrots, nectarines, cucumbers and co-conuts are all excellent for flushing the system and repairing the cells and organs. Some of these items may have to be processed with a food processor first before they can be juiced. It is im-portant that you do not cook any of these fruits or vegetables before juicing them. Temperatures over 112 degrees will kill the enzymes present in the foods you plan to juice. The enzymes are necessary for the juicing to be beneficial. By trial and error, you will determine what small appliance to use for the different produce. For example, bananas should not be processed in a juicer or food processor. They do well in a blender. Usually the fruit with high water contents do better in a juicer, whereas fruit or vegetables that are more meatier do better in a blender or food processor. Experience will teach you

A word of warning about the juicing of watermelon in particular and melons in general. Watermelons should not be mixed with juices from other fruits and vegetables. The combination will cause stomach problems due to the fact that melons are so high in water that the enzymes in them breakdown the food ultra fast. When combined with fruits and vegetables that transit the system slower, the decomposing melons mix with the predigested foods and cause stomach aches and discomfort including headaches in some people! It is safe to mix the melon varieties together though.

When we do our juice fast, we make sure that we allow the poisons and toxins to continue to flow out, by visiting the toilet often. Daily we empty the waste from our systems. If we find that we are not regular or impacted or clogged in anyway, we drink a cup of senna pod herbal tea to soften the stool, so it will flow out freely. Either senna pod or cascara sagrada teas are both excellent as colon flushes. The main thing to remember is that the waste that is brought down in the system by juicing should exit the system immediately. You must keep yourself regular. In the beginning, when we first started this regimen, we were more impacted, so it was necessary to assist the body in eliminating. After doing the process for awhile you will see that it is much easier for your body to flush itself. It is fiber in the diet that helps us all to stay regular anyway, so when you juice fast you are not taking in much fiber therefore your body may need the herbal tea boost. The teas should be drunk without sweeteners, however if you must use a sweetener don't use any chemical sweetener nor sugar. Maple syrup, honey, agave or Stevia would be good choices. Especially if you are diabetic be careful, however Stevia has been used by diabetics without any problem.

For those people that have severe intestinal blockage, like those who eliminate maybe once a week or every two weeks, you could have a professional colonic done. Your system is extremely clogged and juicing will only bring down more waste that will need to be eliminated. A colonic machine is an apparatus that uses warm water or a special saline solution to flush your system as you view what comes out of you. It is done by a specialist in clinical setting and it is considered safe and very beneficial for severely impacted people.

Another option, although not quite as effective, is to give yourself an enema, in the privacy of your own home. This is what we chose to do. Enema kits can be purchased at any health food store. When we do an enema, we use organically grown coffee instead of purified water, because it is much more effective in ridding the body of waste. The caffeine in the coffee is absorbed by the liver and gallbladder, further strengthening their functions. We also use sodium bicarbonate or baking soda. Purified water with herbal solutions are also good, and can be just as effective. In the back of the book, I will give more instructions on taking enemas. If you have a chronic disease such as cancer of any of the internal organs and especially the intestines, colon or rectum, it is not wise to give yourself an enema nor have a colonic done. Consult your physician concerning this.

Key points outlined in chapter

(1)

(2)

(3)

(4)

(5)

Changes I can make to improve my health

(1)

(2)

(3)

(4)

(5)

CHAPTER EIGHT
THE RIGHT FOODS – THE HEALING

LIVE OR DEAD FOODS – WHICH DO YOU PREFER?

If you are eating a plant base diet, then all of your foods are still alive when you consume them. A healthy body will be a body that is nourished properly on a daily basis. Only live foods can deliver the proper nutrients to nourish the body. Dead foods automatically deliver poisons because anything that has died has begun a stage called decomposition or decay. At this writing I am not a vegan nor even vegetarian, although I have been in my life. I mention this fact because I am both ministering to you as well as myself. It does not make much sense to poison ones own body, then wonder why you are in bad health. Nobody force feeds us. We willingly choose to eat death rather than life. It gives all of us something to think about. If you eat an apple, its' seed is still alive to produce after its' kind. Until you bake your potato, it can be sprouted to produce more potatoes. Your beans and peas can be sprouted. Even your grains can be sprouted. Because all of these foods are still alive they are nutrient dense and are provided by God to rejuvenate our systems. "You are what you eat", is an old saying that many of us have heard, but do we believe it. If you eat death, you will die, especially if you eat predominantly dead foods on a consistent basis. The eating of dead foods is a progressive death sentence. Many people say they can't stand vegetables or anything green. Many people never eat fruit. I personally know these people myself. Many people are heavy meat eaters and they feel they must have some meat with every meal. I had a supervisor who was one of the nicest men I have ever met. He use to call me the rabbit because for every lunch I would have a salad or something fresh, green and alive. He mainly ate meat. I was sadden at his funeral, but he chose to go out, with his meat! In an earlier chapter of this book, I mentioned Hippocrates, who was the father of modern medicine. One of his famous quotes was " let your food be your medicine and let your medicine be your food". Do you realize that if he were alive today that this statement could very well cost him his medical license. The AMA would not be happy with such a statement.

Lets talk about fresh fruits and vegetables for a moment and their benefit to the human body. Usually when I say fresh, I mean organic, although some locally grown produce are actually fresh. Some of this information will be a review for you, but I will endeavor to point out some important aspects that were not mentioned earlier. When the supermarkets talk about fresh they usually mean fresh in appearance, texture or even smell. If fruits and vegetables didn't appear to be fresh in the stores, you obviously would not purchase them. It is for this reason that preservatives are used to make the fruits and vegetables appear fresher. There are different methods employed by companies to make their produce appear fresh.

Some fruits and or vegetables are sprayed with sulfur dioxide, some with methylcyclopropene and some with methyl bromide. I am sure that these chemicals have some side effects, which is why it is a good idea to wash all fruit and vegetables before consuming them. Any organically grown produce will not be sprayed with anything and therefore not have a long shelf life. When we buy our produce we make sure that it will be used within a few days at the most because even if refrigerated, it will not stay crisp and fresh long. If your produce begins to lose the crispness, remember they still can be juiced. The shelf life of organic foods will be one thing you definitely notice that differentiates it from non organic foods. The main thing and most important will be the taste. Have you ever wondered why food use to taste so good, in the good old days? One reason is that the foods you grew up on were a lot more organic and usually were locally grown and the soil was healthy. The taste of organic food will amaze you. The difference between a regular supermarket hybrid tomato and an organic heirloom tomato is about as vast as the taste between a apple and a cucumber. They actually taste like two different food items. Another thing to note is that the chemicals added to produce also change the taste.

We need to understand the importance of the term locally grown. If you are in an area where you just cannot find organic produce, then by all means buy locally grown produce. Although not superior to organic, many locally grown products have less chemical additives, preservatives and pesticide contamination. Much chemical contamination of foods occur because of the time frame associated with the harvest to market process and the required transportation. If a product is grown on the other side of the world, then something obviously must be done to preserve some of its' quality. We as consumers have ourselves to blame for this problem. We are the ones who demand that the stores supply watermelons in December or peaches in January. It all boils down to supply and demand. If you just have to have what you want when you want it, you will pay the price. Most people who are concerned about their health, eat what is in season at any given time. This is another reason why locally grown produce is good. There are some foods that are grown in greenhouses or indoors in controlled environments, which allows them to be grown during anytime of the year. In most cases this is done by people on their own who have taken control of their lives and have their own gardens. An important point to remember. Some locally grown or home grown products are organic, but without the certification a person can not say that their product is organic. It is a matter of money! It can cost thousands of dollars to get and maintain a certification. Depending on your relationship with your supplier, they may tell you that they use no pesticides, herbicides or poisons in anyway. At the local farmer's markets you can establish a relationship with your supplier and it is a good thing to do.

Briefly I will address another so-called food group and that is meats. I say so-called because the foods in this group actually do more harm than good. If you are a meat eater, there are some important things you should know. Limit the size of your portions to 4 oz. or less per meal. Don't consume meat at every meal. Don't fry your meats because of the added fat. You are already eating too much fat in consuming the meat, so don't add more fat on top of it. Although it may taste great, pork because of the nature of the animal, is not the best meat to eat. Chew or masticate your meat thoroughly before swallowing, because it takes a long time for meat to digest. You really overwork your enzymes and digestive system when you eat meat. It may take days to fully digest and in some cases never gets fully digested. It is best to eat your fruits or vegetables before the meat because of the digestion time and don't wash your meat down with liquids. I've said enough about meat in previous chapters, so I think you realize the potential dangers, so be cautious.

As far as dairy is concerned, we humans are the only animal in the world that need milk after adolescence. Another thing that amazes me is that we are the only species of animal that thrive on another species' milk. There are organizations that encourage new mothers not to breast feed, yet promote the consumption of another species' milk. Scientist have proved that the immune system of breast feed infants are much stronger than those raised on formulas or cows' milk. After you are weaned from your mothers' breast, you do not need anymore milk in your life. After our sons were weaned from my wife's breast, we never gave them milk again and they have been pictures of health their entire lives. You can get all the calcium you need from vegetables. This fact may not do much for the profits of the dairy associations, but it is true.

The next food group is important and that is the grains. A diet high in whole grains makes the body stronger and adds necessary fiber to help with elimination. Whole grain foods are associated with a significantly lower risk of developing cardiovascular diseases, including heart disease and stroke. Also they lessens the onset of obesity and diabetes. There are many grains that are not popular in the Western world, that are very beneficial to our bodies. Many people are not aware of quinoa, amaranth, buckwheat (which is not actually a grain), millet, spelt, farro and there are others. Give them a try and discover new taste and nutrition. When you eat rice, make sure it is not white rice because white rice has very little, if any, nutritional content. Brown rice or wild rice are much better. The same thing goes for the eating of white breads. If you must eat bread, eat whole grain breads. White bread is also void of nutrients and should not be eaten. White bread when eaten turns into a sticky substance like Elmer's glue in your intestine. Many products that have been stripped of nutrition are then fortified with nutrients. This is important to remember, if a product is labeled fortified with vitamins, it is not wholesome because reintroducing nutrients to a product that has previously been stripped of nutrients does not work! It upsets the nutritional balance of the product and actually does more harm than good.

While on the subject of whole grains, for years nutritionist have been advocating whole grain wheat for consumption. BEWARE OF THE DANGERS OF WHEAT! This current wheat is a completely different strain of wheat than the wheat consumed by our grand parents and great grand parents. This hybrid form of wheat has been selectively bred and it is not even remotely close to the wheat consumed in past generations. This current wheat crop stands only about 2 ½ feet tall in contrast to its' predecessor which was 4-5 feet in height. The differences don't stop there. Although initially grown to curtail world hunger by increasing the yield, which it successfully did, this new wheat is extremely dangerous to our health. From research done by Dr.

Mark Hyman, Dr. William Davis and others, we have evidence to prove that this current wheat product differs in three main ways.

1. It contains a super starch – Amylopectin A that is super fattening.

2. It contains a form of super gluten that is super inflammatory – triggering toxicity.

3. It contains forms of a super toxic drug that is super addictive making a person crave and eat more.

This wheat is worst than sugar. Two slices of whole wheat bread is equivalent to 6 teaspoons of sugar and the real kicker is that wheat is in virtually every product we buy in the supermarkets. I will give a list of just some of those products, mind you there are many more. All breads, whether wheat or not, cereals, crackers, all pastries, including cakes and pies, pizza, breaded or battered foods, canned soups, frozen or canned vegetables, dips & gravies, sauces, salad dressings, pasta, ground spices, instant drinks like coffee, tea or cocoa, desserts – ice cream, sherbert, prepared/packaged meats, pasteurized cheese, beer, candy, chewing gum, etc. From this list it is obvious that it is virtually impossible to avoid wheat completely, but you can make some changes.

From a health point of view, this new wheat has been medically linked to the following diseases and conditions, celiac disease, acid diseases, acidosis, acid reflex, constant feelings of hunger, cramps, lupus, obesity, diabetes, heart disease, osteoporosis, leaky gut syndrome, increase blood glucose, chronic diarrhea, rheumatoid arthritis, fatigue, joint pain, swollen legs, colon abnormalities, etc. When you try to eliminate wheat from your diet, you will go through withdrawals, which can range from anxiety, depression, irritability, headaches, insomnia, etc. and these conditions can last for a week or more. I realize that most people will not grow and process their own food or not eat at restaurants to avoid the wheat problems, but you do need to know why you are not feeling well or why you may have a particular disease or condition. AVOID WHEAT AS MUCH AS YOU CAN AND READ YOUR LABELS. To find out more about this interesting discovery, I have listed both Dr. Davis and Dr. Hyman's books in the suggested reading section.

Another important food group is nuts, which are full of vitamins, minerals, natural fats and oils. In fact the oils that are in nuts help with the good cholesterol in the body. Nuts are really the seed of dried fruits. The shells being the dried fruit that has dried on the tree. Nuts are high in omega 3 oils, a good source of fiber, reduce the risk of heart problems and are beneficial to diabetic patients. One study said that two to three years could be added to the life of a person who consumed nuts on a regular basis. They are a very high source of energy also and most Americans have little or no energy.

FOOD PREPARATION
Now that you know the right foods to eat, you need to know how to prepare them. The best preparation is no preparation. What I mean by that is you should eat your fruits and vegetables raw for the most wholesome nutritious benefit. Your body was designed to eat raw foods. Remember when vegetables are heated above 112 degrees, the nutritional content will be virtually destroyed and the enzymes in the food will be affected. If you must cook your vegetables to get them down, then steam them or saute them. The section on recipes will give you some ideas on how to prepare raw vegetables. They are very good that way, if they are prepared and combined properly. Many African Americans still eat the traditional soul food dishes,

which they were raised on. Many soul food vegetable dishes are over cooked and the nutrients are destroyed in the food item. If your vegetables are dull in color and not bright, they have been overcooked. Watch for crispness, vegetables should remain crisp. The color of your vegetables will get brighter if cooked slightly. Raw is still the best and healthiest way to go. Fruit should be eaten raw also and selected if possible at the peak of ripeness. If your fruit is picked and eaten while fully ripe, the sugar content and nutritional value will be at its' peak. Another thing to remember about ripe fruit, the enzymes in the fruit has already began to breakdown the food, which makes it easier for you to digest your fruit. With organic fruits, this is evident because a good organic farmer will know when to pick and deliver the best product to market. However non organic fruit, especially when it is not locally grown, will be picked before it ripens. This process causes the fruit to be void of most of it's potential nutritional content. Fruit is picked before ripening so it can withstand the long travel time before it reaches the market. Another reason for picking the fruit before it is ripe is so it will be hard enough to withstand the transportation without getting bruised. Fruit grown and picked by utilizing this process is harder to digest, thereby overworking your enzymes also. You only have so many enzymes, so use them judiciously.

Since meat eaters should not fry their meats, the following methods of cooking are safer. The best methods to use is to broil, boil or bake. The eating of raw or very rare meat is not advisable, because of the potential parasite infestation or bacterial contamination. If the meat is prepared in one of the methods mentioned, the oils can drain out of the meat to minimize the amount of fats you ingest. Never eat meat that is not thoroughly cooked!

SPROUTING

While we are on the subject of food preparation, I will discuss the value of sprouting. Sprouting is a great way to get the most nutrients from grains, beans, peas or seeds. Many people buy sprouts but it is a lot easier and more cost effective to sprout your own foods. Before I explain how to sprout, lets look at the value of sprouting. The vitamins, minerals and nutrients are packed into the grains, beans, peas or seeds and when they germinate or sprout, supercharged nutrients are immediately released like an explosion. So sprouting allows you to get the most out of that food item before time, processing and cooking minimizes the nutritional potency. Another fact about sprouting is that a little goes a long way. For example, 5 Tablespoons full of alfalfa seeds cost about $0.25, yet it will yield about 1 lb. of alfalfa sprouts. This is a quite a savings over the cost in the health food stores. Sprouts are a whole lot easier to digest than the grain, bean, pea or seed that they come from. Your body can utilize the nutrients immediately. From experiments scientist have discovered that the nutritional content of the sprouted product is 2 – 3 times greater. For optimal nutrition sprout as many food items as possible. Sprouting can be done right in your own kitchen. You can buy sprouting kits at your local health food store. To start with you can use any jar with a lid, like a 1-quart mason jar. Cut a piece of screen out large enough to cover the mouth of the jar, making sure you can still screw on the top. Put your grains, beans, peas or seeds in and cover them with purified or distilled water. Don't put too many in the jar, just about 15 Tablespoons of food. Let the jar sit in the kitchen for about 24 hours then drain the water, rinse the product then turn the jar upside down in the dish drain at a 45 degree angle so air can flow in. This part of the process works better if covered with a dish towel or dish rag so that it is dark for the first 6-8 hours, then every 6 – 8 hours drain and rinse and continue this process until you see the product split open and start sprouting. Depending on what you are sprouting, it may take anywhere from 2 – 5 days. Just keep checking and rinsing so that the water does not get stagnant. When the seed splits open you will see a little tail start to grow then the first leaves developing. You can use them at any stage you like for snacking, salads, sandwiches, soups or garnishes. Try sprouting some sunflower seeds, they are my favorite! The seeds or nuts must be raw and unsalted.

Key points outlined in chapter

(1)

(2)

(3)

(4)

(5)

Changes I can make to improve my health

(1)

(2)

(3)

(4)

(5)

CHAPTER NINE
JUICING YOUR WAY TO HEALTH

This may be one of the most important chapters in this book, although it is a short one. In this chapter I will reveal to you how you can undo or remedy years of abuse inflicted on your body from unhealthy eating practices and the consumption of toxic drugs. What is so awesome about this method, is the fact that it can be done in a very short time by anyone. In this instant society that we live in, where people have very little to no patience, this easy method should make anyone happy. The key to reversing your health dilemmas, is through juicing or more accurately juice fasting. It may be called juice fasting, juice feasting or juice cleansing, but whatever you want to call it, it is basically the same thing. Your meals each day consist of only fruits and vegetables in juice form. The reason this is so effective is that you can consume an enormous amount of produce when it is drank as oppose to being eaten. The benefit with juicing is that you actually overload your nutrient starved system with enough nutrients to aid in both flushing the system of waste, chemicals, poisons, toxins and unwanted fats and you begin the building of new cells to maintain a healthy system.

The fruit juices cleanse and flush your system and the vegetable juices build and repair cellular systems. This double action also causes your body to heal from illnesses, disorders and diseases, while you lose weight. It is a win win situation for your body. As you should have learned by now, the body is designed by God to repair itself, if given the opportunity to do so. The juice fast gives your body that opportunity and the body can cleanse and repair itself in an unbelievably short amount of time. We have found that the best method for us is to have fruit juice in the morning as a liquid breakfast with protein powder and a lunch and diner juice of primarily vegetables with some apple or other sweet fruit to balance the taste. There are no hard and fast rules, but it is better to consume more vegetables so that new cells can be built. The fruit juices are a lot easier to drink of course because they are sweet and we all have our sweet tooth to some extent. Use only organic produce because you have enough toxins in your body already. We like to juice our own because we don't have to worry about any preservatives added to our juice. Another important point is the fact that you can use herbal teas as you juice fast, since they are liquid. We use teas to assist in the flushing and eliminating that our system experiences, during the juicing process. I gave you a list of which fruit and vegetables to eat, those are the same ones you can juice. Many people have experienced weight loss, healed organs and unbelievable health breakthroughs while doing the fast. Just go online to Youtube and key in "juicing"and hear some of the testimonies. You will be amazed! If you are under a doctors' care, discuss it with your doctor by all means, however you are just feeding yourself but doing so without chewing. Remember you will need a juicer, food processor and a blender. Personally I would not do a juice fast until I could make my own juice because the results would be more dramatic. However, if it is impossible for you to juice your own for some reason, just purchase the healthiest juices you possibly can. The main thing is for you to "just do it."

Key points outlined in chapter

(1)

(2)

(3)

(4)

(5)

Changes I can make to improve my health

(1)

(2)

(3)

(4)

(5)

CHAPTER TEN
HERBS AND FOLK MEDICINES

First of all we need to define the word herb. A herb is a seed-producing annual, biennial, or perennial plant that does not develop persistent woody tissue but dies down at the end of a growing season. It also is a plant or plant part valued for its medicinal, savory or aromatic qualities. These are general definitions because some herbs are harder to define. From these dictionary definitions we can see that herbs are plants that produce food, seasonings, medicines and pleasant aromas for olfactory pleasure. A herb therefore can be a root, stem, leaf, flower or fruit, since they all constitute a plant. Remember God said "the leaves of the plant would be for the healing of the nation", and Hippocrates said "your food shall be your medicine and your medicine shall be your food." Why then do herbs get such a negative rap in our country from the media and so-called experts. Well to "kill, steal and destroy," you must first seduce your enemy. Are we being lied to as a nation of people, since over 40% of the drugs on the market were derived from plants (herbs) and chemical compounds in plants (herbs)? Well over 120 compounds were discovered from plants just a decade ago and daily new ones are being found. The reason why the plant itself is not introduced to the public as a cure is because no monetary gain can be realized since a plant cannot be patented!!!

The use of herbs or plants for not only food but medicine actually predates written human history. The farther back you go, the more prevalent was the use of plants as medicines. All of the people groups known today that have avoided Westernization and have remained in isolation from so-called progress, use plants as medicines. A lot of the medical maladies that they do contract are those that have been introduced into their societies by outside influences. Much money today is spent on research in these isolated pockets of the world, to determine what plant is being used and how. My mother and grandmother knew which plants to use to cure all their family ailments. These plants were native to the area they lived in. Much of this knowledge has unfortunately been lost by most family groups. It serves to prove that God has provided for His people. We just need to know which plants are beneficial and for what purpose they are to be used. It was Dale Carnegie who said, "It's a shame that each new generation must find the way to success by trial and error when the principles are really clear-cut." For us in the Body of Christ that is definitely true because God has told us in His Word. When we eat the plants, they not only nourish our bodies but they prevent our bodies from getting sick, help to maintain wellness and cleanse our bodies of waste.

Plants are a complete food source for all aspects of wellness, spirit, soul and body.

Read the first chapter of the book of Daniel in your Bible. In this chapter you will see that Daniel and his friends were opposed to eating the food of their captors because the rich delicacies were not healthy. Although this was food fit for a king, they realized that God had a better dietary plan for their lives. As the story unfolds, we see that a challenge was proposed by Daniel to prove the value of a simple plant based diet and its superiority to rich foods. Daniels' adversary accepted his challenge and after 10 days of eating their plant based diet, they were determined to be more fit, healthy and energetic than their counterparts who ate the kings' cuisine. For those of you who do not see the analogy between us in the Body of Christ and the food provided by this worlds' system, I will explain. We are in this world but not of this world. Read Rom. 12:2; John 17:14 – 17. We cannot expect any aspect of this system to work because it was designed by satan. We are members of a greater kingdom, the Kingdom of God and God has laws that must be obeyed. The Babylonian system is not unlike our system and we in the Body of Christ should respond as Daniel did or at least not be surprised when we suffer for not responding to Gods' mandates or laws. You choose this day whom you will serve. God wants you well so you can live healthy lives that contrast to the lives of others, and as a result the door to evangelize will be open by your lifestyle, which is really your witness.

COMMON HERBS FOR SIMPLE AILMENTS

I will talk initially about the more common herbs but at the end of this chapter I will talk about specific herbs used as cleansers and detoxifiers for serious illnesses and diseases. The following list of herbs are the ones we try to keep in our medicine cabinet for common illnesses and minor ailments. We had these herbs available when our kids were growing up but now we keep them for emergency purposes when our grandchildren are ill or our friends are in need.

AGAVE is a plant that has gained popularity in the last few years in this country due to its nectar, which has been used as a substitute for sugar. The plant also has healing properties. It has been successfully used as a antiseptic, diuretic and laxative.

ALFALFA is known primarily as a form of hay for livestock, but the alfalfa plant is loaded with vitamins and minerals. It has been reported that between alfalfa and kelp virtually every vitamin and mineral known to man is evident. It can be used as a tonic by drinking it, or prepared as a herbal tea.

ALOE is another very popular plant that is gaining more and more respect for its varied uses. Although the juice or pulp of the plant is quite bitter, it can be mixed with other liquids and drank. It has healing properties and is good against any infections. We use it on cuts, bruises and abrasions instead of bandages because it cleans the wound, seals out bacteria and covers the wounds as it hardens. It is natures bandaid. It is good on any skin disorder from simple sunburn to deep cuts as it will stop the bleeding also. It is excellent as a cleanser for the face and hands and also good for your hair when you shampoo or condition. Everyone needs an aloe plant, an especially if you have children. My mother who lived to 95 ½, drank aloevera water daily for the last twenty years of her life. When she died, she had no diseases, was on no medication and was just as sharp as ever. Her longevity was attributed to many factors however, she ate organic vegetables from her garden, she watched what she consumed, she always drank plenty of water, she ate very little meat, never ate junk foods and she refused any prescription drugs with their side effects.

AMARANTH is a plant that is gaining popularity as a grain although it really is not a grain. It is really valued for its' seeds which are excellent tasting and very high in nutritional value. We use it as a cereal in the morning like oatmeal, oat bran or wheat bran. The plant also has medicinal advantages as an astringent if taken orally for diarrhea, dysentery, hemorrhaging from the bowels and excessive menstruation. The leaf of the plant can be eaten in salads.

BLUE VERVAIN OR VERVAIN is a plant that we use often to induce sleep. It is a natural tranquilizer that is good for nervous disorders. It is good for fevers, colds and chest congestion.

CALENDULA is the name of the marigold plant. You all have seen the beautiful golden, yellow, orange, blossoms of this flower. It is a plant that grows wild and is used by gardeners to beautify landscaping. We use the petals of the flower dried and prepared as a tea for gastrointestinal problems like ulcers, stomach cramps, colitis and diarrhea. The plant is highly effective in menstrual difficulties and it can be used as a salve for external wounds. I will tell you how to make your own salves in the following chapter – Herbal Application & Cleansing Techniques

CAMOMILE is a mild herb that we have used for calming our children when they were restless. It is good in flatulent colic and dyspepsia. When made into a rubbing oil, it is good for swellings, callouses and painful joints. I will teach you how to make your own rubbing oils also in the next chapter.

CAYENNE is a pepper plant and there are many different ones. Its main property is capsicum, which gives it a hot characteristic. We all know of its value as a highly prized seasoning, however it is so good for many other things. It is a general stimulant that acts as a tonic to help build up resistance to colds and the flu. It is great for ulcerated stomachs and strengthening the digestive system. Cayenne is very good in removing mucous and phlegm from the mucous membranes in the body. If you seem to always have a cold or know someone who does, start consuming more cayenne. Slowly build up your tolerance, your health will thank you. Too much can lead to gastrointestinal problems and kidney damage, so be aware. The various pepper plants have varying degrees of hotness. The degrees of hotness is determined by the amounts of capsicum or capsaicin in each plant and it is measured by the Scoville scale. The various pepper plants are very effective on sores, bruises, and skin problems when used as a topical treatment.

CHICKWEED is a weed or plant that is found in most lawns and is an excellent addition to any salad or sandwich, used like sprouts or spinach. It is a very delicate and fragile plant. Medicinally it is valued for its laxative properties and its benefit in serious constipation problems. It is also used as an ointment for bruises, irritations and skin problems.

COMFREY is another very useful herb that many households used for years. It has been used for throat inflammations, hoarseness, and bleeding gums. It is also good for digestive and stomach problems, for intestinal difficulties, for excessive menstrual flow, bloody urine, diarrhea, gastro-intestinal ulcers, dysentery, and persistent coughs. Externally it is beneficial in wounds, bruises, sores, and insect bites. It is truly an amazing plant that has a myriad of uses.

DANDELION although considered a weed by most people, is an excellent plant for its iron content. When you were a kid, I'm sure you picked up dandelion stems with their ball of seeds and blew them all away. That is the dandelion plant. It has leaves that are excellent for salads and are even sold in the better health food stores. Why buy it when you can pick it anywhere. Knowledge is what God said His people were destroyed for a lack of. When the leaves of the dandelion plant are dried, they can be made into a tea that is not only a great source of extra iron but one of the best blood builders and purifiers you can take. Why buy Geritol or SSS tonic when you can make a pot of dandelion tea for yourself and get all the iron you need.

ECHINACEA is one of the most powerful blood-purifying plants used for conditions such as acne, eczema and boils. It promotes proper digestion and is excellent in fevers. Since many people are afraid of fevers, I might add that they are a good thing because your body is letting you know that it has been compromised in some way, form or fashion. It is natures alarm, telling us that there is a problem and something is not right. Eliminate the problem and the fever will dissipate. Echinacea is excellent in such cases.

FENUGREEK is one of the oldest medicinal plants used by man, dating back to the early Egyptians and Hippocrates. Aside from its culinary uses it was also used as an expectorant to rid the system of mucous and phlegm in the throat, esophagus, lungs and bronchial tubes. When made into a poultice it was very successful against gouty pain, sciatica, swollen glands, wounds, tumors, sores and skin irritations. I will explain in the next chapter how to make a homemade poultice.

GINGER is an indigenous plant to tropical Asia. The root of the plant is what is used in many oriental dishes. It has a strong pungent taste and smell and is quite hot when eaten alone. It is an excellent food, with an unusual but distinct taste. From a medicinal point of view it is highly prized in Oriental medicine. It promotes cleansing of the system through perspiration. It is said to be good in suppressed menstruation. It is very good when used as a gargle for sore throats and in fevers or colds. It acts as an expectorant to rid the body of mucous and soothes the membranes.

GINSENG is another Asiatic plant that is used extensively by the Oriental in their medicines. Ginseng has a wide variety of uses and has proven to be very effective in most conditions. For thousands of years the Chinese have considered this plant as a panacea for practically all ailments. The Chinese almost have a love affair with this plant and it is considered an integral part of their culture. It is a stimulant and has been used for inflammatory illnesses, hemorrhages, blood diseases, normalizing menstruation, easing childbirth, promoting appetite, helping digestive disorders, stimulant for the central nervous system and various glands, coughs, colds, chest problems and even as an aphrodisiac.

While on the subject of the Chinese, for years their medical practices operated on the premise that they only got paid when the patient was cured. There are still a handful of doctors who abide by this ancient practice. Another very important point about their medical practices was the fact that they looked for the cause of the illnesses and tried to correct the causes as opposed to their western counterparts who only deal with symptoms.

GOLDENSEAL is a herb we have used often for colds, symptoms of colds, sore throats, congestion and swollen tonsils, when drank as a tea. Sniff the powder up the nasal passage for nasal congestion. It is good as an antiseptic mouthwash. It is very effective as a solution for a vaginal douche. It has been used in many homes as a laxative and for stomach ailments.

HYSSOP is one of our favorite herbs. We probably use more hyssop than any other herb. All households should keep this herb handy. It is an old herb mentioned on several occasions in the Old Testament of the Holy Bible. It was used in biblical days as a cleanser for the body. We use it to break up congestion in the throat and chest cavity. When no other herb seems to be effective, hyssop will always do the job. If taken in tea form, it will soothe the symptoms associated with colds. It is considered to be a very potent herd and should not be used haphazardly. We have used it quite judiciously over the years with no problems.

MULLEIN is one of the great sleep inducing herbs. However the sleep is a tranquil sleep not like the herb Valerian, which I will discuss later. Mullein soothes the nerves and brings a calming effect to the system. A tea made from the leaves is also good in any respiratory problems like colds, sore throats, hoarseness, congestion and coughing. The flower of the plant has been known to relieve pain and is useful for external applications with wounds, sores, warts and any skin problems.

NETTLE is another very popular old remedy that was used in many households prior to the prescription drug era. Nettle is useful in many different conditions. Before I list its medicinal value, I will point out its use in salads, especially if the younger plants are used, the older plants can be harmful if eaten. Fresh juice from the plant has been used to stimulate the digestive system and promote milk flow in nursing mothers. As a tea it is useful if blood is in the urine, helpful with hemorrhoidal conditions, urinary tract problems, diarrhea and menstrual complications. The tea used externally is beneficial in hair loss also.

OLIVE is a very well known and used plant, especially the fruit of the tree. Of course olive oil is one of the most beneficial oils in use for both cooking, eating and external application for skin and hair. Many people are not aware of the fact that the leaves and bark of the tree are used for medicinal purposes. The leaves and inner bark are a great natural antiseptic and are used in fevers and helpful in nervous tension to relieve stress, almost like a tranquilizer. The oil acts as a mild laxative and is helpful to the mucous membranes and is reported to dissolve cholesterol. Externally the oil of the olive is good for burns, bruises, insect bites and intense itching. The oil is used as a base in the making of salves, ointments and liniments. This is one of the oldest plants in the world.

RED CLOVER is a wonderful herb used for quieting the nerves and inducing sound sleep. It is a great blood purifier. It is one of natures greatest plants to fight cancerous growths and tumors. It is good in any skin eruption, sores and wounds. It is a wonderful herb to be used by women with fibroid tumors and any uterine conditions. It can be prepared as a vaginal douche.

ROSEMARY is a wonderful seasoning herb and is a great aromatic. It is an antispasmodic and stimulant and as such is helpful in promoting liver function, the production of bile and proper digestion. Rosemary can raise the blood pressure and it improves the circulation. When combined with other herbs it has proven beneficial in external applications. A tea of this herb makes an excellent mouthwash and it is good for halitosis.

SAGE is another herb that is good used externally and internally. Sage is of course an excellent seasoning with a hardy strong flavor. It is used often in Italian cuisines. A tea from the herb is good in nervous conditions, trembling, depression and vertigo. As a gargle it is good for sore throats, laryngitis and tonsillitis. Externally sage is good as a hair rinse and is good for dry scalp and dandruff. There are different varieties of sage, however they are all beneficial and easy to grow or pick it in the wild.

SAW PALMETTO is a herb that has become popular in the treatment of men with prostrate problems, usually enlarged. It is also useful in all diseases of the reproductive organs, ovaries and the male testicles.
While on the subject of enlarged prostrates, the deficiency of zinc is the main culprit because of the poor soil condition in this country, zinc is almost nonexistent. It is reported that most men in their fifties should expect to have enlarged prostates, however it is not something men have to settle for or look forward to. When you switch to organic foods, which have a much higher zinc content, the prostrate size will diminish. Many of the issues men deal with concerning impotency, premature ejaculation and related symptoms can be directly linked to poor diet. Improve your diet and you will improve your performance. It is as simple as that. The only reason the problem is accepted

in men at that age is because most men eat the Standard American Diet (SAD). Have you ever thought about how much money is made from male enhancement products? Many companies are glad men have these issues!

Back to the benefits of Saw Palmetto. The herb is useful in all kinds of throat troubles, especially when there is excessive mucous discharge from the head and nose, good in treatment of colds, bronchitis, la grippe, whooping cough and where the throat is irritated and painful.

SENNA or Senna Pod is an excellent laxative that will relieve the intestines even when there is impaction. The pods actually breakdown the fecal matter into particles that can more easily be discharged from the colon. There can be griping associated with the herb, especially as it is working in your system on the waste matter, however this can be minimized by diluting the herb with much water. The herb is also good in ridding the system of parasitic worms, that have been killed by the juicing. Practically all Americans have worms whether you believe me or not. I would venture to guess that at least 90% of Americans have at least one type of parasite in their system and there are many type. It was said by Dr. Frank Nova, Chief of the Laboratory for Parasitic Disease (National Institute of Health), "There are more parasitic infections acquired in this country than in Africa." If you have never addressed this condition in your body, you need to! Many of you who are suffering with fatigue problems can attribute the fatigue to the presence of parasites in your system, especially if you eat a lot of meat and have never been dewormed. Senna Pod tea is made by soaking 8-12 pods in water for 12 hours.

VALERIAN is one of the most effective sleep inducing herbs.

When no other herb will work, VALERIAN will cause you to sleep. It will put you into such a deep sleep that it is wise to minimize its use until you have determined your systems tolerance of the herb. It is considered a nerve tonic – very quieting and soothing. It has been used when people were hysterical, to calm them down. It will promote menstruation, help in measles, colds, congestion, convulsions in infants, heart palpitation, to relieve gas, to break up gravel in the bladder and help ulcerated stomachs. This herb can also be applied externally for sores and pimples. We keep a supply of this herb handy because of its' varied use.

The following list of herbs are used when doing a cleansing or detoxifying. Some of them have been mentioned before because herbs have varied uses, however, aside from their other uses they all have been used successfully to rid the body of waste, chemicals, poisons, toxins and excessive fats.

DANDELION
MILK THISTLE
CASCARA SAGRADA
SENNA
LICORICE ROOT
PSYLLIUM SEED
ALFALFA
YUCCA ROOT
VIOLET LEAF
GUARGUM
MARSHMALLOW ROOT
BLACK WALNUT HULL
PUMPKIN SEEDS
IRIS MOSS

PASSION FLOWER LEAF
WITCH HAZEL
CAPSCACIN
GENTIAN ROOT
CRANBERRY
HORSETAIL
SLIPPERY ELM BARK
MULLEIN LEAF
BLACK COHOSH
BURDOCK ROOT
ECHINACEA
FENNEL SEED
GINGER
PAPAYA
CINNAMON
CAYENNE
DEVIL'S CLAW
FENUGREEK
GOLDENSEAL ROOT

MASTER TONIC

Another healthy product my wife and I take is a tonic called
Master tonic. This is a tonic that was first introduced by the famous Paul C. Bragg, N.D., Ph.D. We make our own and try to
drink it daily. When I was a kid my mother use to give us health
tonics several times during the year to keep us healthy and able
to fight off sicknesses. This is a similar tonic. It is made up of 5
of best antioxidants known to man, onions, garlic, ginger, hot
peppers and horseradish in a liquid base of Braggs' Apple Cider
Vinegar. It is made by grinding and grating 1 lb. of each of the
ingredients, then immersing them in the vinegar and letting
concoction sit for at least two weeks. The longer it sits, the

stronger the tonic gets. Afterward you can drain off the liquid and drink 1-2 tablespoons daily. Keep the pulp or residue because it can be chewed if you ever have a sore throat or any respiratory condition and within minutes relief will come. This tonic and the pulp can last indefinitely, if kept refrigerated or in a cool place. Try it and you will probably never get sick again. We have been making this tonic for about 6-7 years and during that time neither me nor my wife have been ill with anything! We have not even had a single cold during that time period. It is important to note that this is arguably one of the most potent anticancer tonics you could take!!!

Key points outlined in chapter

(1)

(2)

(3)

(4)

(5)

Changes I can make to Improve my health

(1)

(2)

(3)

(4)

(5)

CHAPTER ELEVEN
THE NUTRITION - MENTAL ILLNESS LINK

As you have probably concluded by now, there are also mental illnesses that have been linked to malnutrition or poor nutrition. It is hard to believe that a country like ours could possibly have a malnutrition problem, the reality is we really have a malnutrition epidemic. Our problem does not necessarily stem from the lack of food but more from the lack of quality nutritious food. "Since many diseases are known to be the result of wrong balance of essential nutrients in the body, adjusting the diet, eliminating junk foods, and ingesting large doses of essential vitamins, minerals, trace metals, amino acids, and polyunsaturated fats, can correct the chemical imbalances of disease." This quote was from a book entitled, Nutrition and Mental Illness - An Orthomolecular Approach to Balancing Body Chemistry by Carl C. Pfeiffer, Ph.D., M.D. This statement echoes the same sentiments that I have been addressing. We are stuffing ourselves with empty calories, or foods that bloat us but do not feed us. This is one of the primary causes of obesity in America and of course serious and chronic diseases.

As my wife an I talk or council with people concerning their health dilemmas, some common statements are echoed. "I don't think I could do that," "but how does it taste?", "I don't think I could eat like that," "I don't have the time to eat that way" or "I don't have the energy to prepare my food properly." These are the responses or excuses most frequently made. The one thing that all the excuses have in common, is the fact that mentally the people are not focused enough on the seriousness of their situations, nor the repercussions of continued bad choices. I am not saying that these people have mental issues but what I am saying is for someone to not be concerned with the quality of their life and how they will exit this life, seem somewhat strange to me!

Before I list some of the mental health diseases that have been directly attributed to poor nutrition, malnutrition or an imbalanced nutritional state, I would like to quote another interesting statement from Dr. Pfeiffer. "There is little doubt nutritional and biochemical imbalances play a large part in behavior disorders. We know of at least nine biochemical imbalances that can result in violent behavior." In light of his statement and the research that he has done, it seems strange that we can still wonder why we have such a crime problem in America and why many of our youth are also so violent? After I list these diseases, I will discuss the common link that most of them have with each other. You might be surprise to know that basically there are three or four nutrient deficiencies that link the diseases that will be outlined.

Alcoholism
Alzheimer
Anxiety
Autism
Depression
Drug Addiction
Extreme Fear
Epilepsy
Hallucination
Insomnia

Mental Retardation
Migraine Headaches
Multiple Sclerosis
Obsession
Paranoia
Phobias
Senility
Schizophrenia
Suicidal Tendency

It is hard to believe that the proper nutrition can help and or cure the above list of diseases but it is a fact and people are being cured daily with the proper megadoses of vitamins, minerals and trace minerals. How can you give yourself a megadose of the right nutrients? I'm glad you asked because as I stated earlier fruit and vegetable juicing is the only way. You could not possibly eat enough fruits and vegetables in one sitting to get the amount of nutrients needed to correct and or eliminate diseases of deficiency. However through juicing, it can be done and done quickly. The only other way is to have a medical practioner inject you with megadoses of the proper deficient nutrients.

In order to overcome these and other health diseases and ailments, you will need to make some drastic changes in your lifestyles. I am not saying you have to go on a diet, you need to make changes because diets are temporary and that is the reason they don't work. Lifestyle changes are everlasting and are needed to reverse some of the illnesses and to live an abundant life of divine health. In the Bible, many times after Jesus prayed and delivered the masses, He would tell them to "go and sin no more." The statement "go and sin no more," implies that the condition He delivered them from was in someway brought on by their own sinful choices. I am telling you that many of your diseases have been brought on by your own choices and by the fact that you have entrusted your health concerns and problems to those who could care less about you personally. God does care about all of us and He wants us to live in divine health. I hope that through this book you will begin to make some serious changes that will lead to a long and healthy life, as my wife and I have done.

By eating a balanced diet of fruits, vegetables, grains, nuts, etc., and juicing often you can live a healthful and long life. You will need to eliminate the bad items from your diet though! By eating properly your body will get the right combination of nutrients in the proper ratio to facilitate divine health. The Creator has placed all the necessary nutrients in the foods for you in the proper combination and ratio, if those food items are grown properly and delivered to you in a timely manner. God is a good God.

Now about those nutrients found lacking in the bodies of those people studied, who had the mental disorders - Magnesium, Manganese, Chromium and Vitamin C, were found in limited amounts in the patients, much below the minimum daily requirements, however Zinc and B6 were almost lacking completely. I want to address the Zinc and B6 connection because it is so vitally important in mental illness and also in other diseases as well.

Zinc is an essential mineral found in every cell of the body. We need Zinc to keep the immune system functioning properly, for blood clotting and for thyroid and reproduction system functions. Our senses of smell, taste and sight are also dependent on proper amounts of Zinc. There is one key factor mentioned and that is the fact that the immune system is compromised. A compromised immune system means that the body is not able to fight off illnesses and the white blood cells can't attack them properly, when they are detected.

B6 is a part of the Vitamin B complex and is essential as a co-enzyme which works with the enzymes to breakdown and use amino acids in the body. B6 plays a role in the creation of antibodies in the immune system that deal with nerve functions. A lack of this vitamin can lead to confusion and irritability. Another key point mentioned in conjunction with B6 is the fact that the immune system again is under attack!

When given megadoses of Zinc and B6, the patients all improved dramatically. How can you personally get megadoses of these nutrients into your system? Juicing can deliver the magadoses needed to your system. I have included a list of the products that contain these two important nutrients. The list will include some items that are not suited for juicing but they should be added to your diet.

Zinc – Avocados, Blackberries, Dates, Loganberries, Pomegranates, Raspberries, Napa Cabbage, Asparagus, Brussels Sprouts, Lima Beans, Okra, Peas, Potatoes, Pumpkins, Shiitake Mushrooms, Spinach and Swiss Chard.

B6 – Avocados, Bananas, Dates, Grapes, Guavas, Mangoes, Pineapples, Pomegranates, Watermelons, Amaranth, Bok Choy, Broccoli, Brussels Sprouts, Butternut Squash, Beans, Green

Peppers, Kale, Lima Beans, Okra, Potatoes, Spinach, Squash, Sweet Potatoes, Pumpkin seeds, Pistacios, Black eyed Peas, Sunflower seeds, Walnuts, Brown rice and Brewers' Yeast.

Key points outlined in chapter

(1)

(2)

(3)

(4)

(5)

Changes I can make to improve my health

(1)

(2)

(3)

(4)

(5)

CHAPTER TWELVE
HERBAL APPLICATION & CLEANSING
TECHNIQUES

In this chapter I will outline some of the herbal application techniques that we use to improve and maintain our families' health condition. I will tell you how to make herbal teas, salves, ointments, rubbing oils and poultices. At the end of the chapter I will explain the proper way to give yourself a enema and also list some of the liquids we use to flush our systems.

Herbal teas are made differently depending on what part of the plant or herb you are going to use. If you are preparing a tea made of either the flower or leaf of the plant then you will boil your water first, put in your tea, cover and just let it simmer in the water with the burner off. The longer the herbs simmer, the stronger the tea. Most teas will be made with one teaspoon of herb to 16 oz. of water. Make sure you use filtered, distilled, purified or natural spring water. Never use faucet water. To sweeten your teas if desired, use any natural sweetener but never sugar or an artificial sweetener. If you are a diabetic, it is best to use Stevia as a sweetener. If you are using the stems or roots of the plant or herb, it is best to put your flame on low after the water has boiled and the herb is placed in. You can cook the herb on a low flame for about 5-10 minutes then cover and let it simmer. The plant parts should be soften so that the pulp is exposed.

To make salves from your herbs, determine whether you want a light salve or heavier salve. Depending on which type you want, you will use slightly different ingredients. The first thing you need to do is make your tea, following the above instructions but make sure you let it sit until it actually cools. This will allow it to get very strong or potent, which is best for salves. Do not strain your tea!! You will need about ½ oz. of beeswax shavings. For a heavier salve use cold press olive oil about 1 ½ cup, for a lighter oil use extra virgin olive oil and ¾ cup of cocoa butter or shea butter. You can use all beeswax if you desire or a combination of shea butter and beeswax. Some people use petroleum jelly or lard instead of beeswax. You still will need the olive oil or cocoanut oil as a substitute.
In a double boiler, cook the oil (olive or cocoanut) and herbal tea together for 3-5 hours. Afterward strain the mixture through a piece of cheesecloth, until you have all the liquid collected. While that is cooling combine the beeswax and shea or cocoa butter in a sauce pan and heat until it blends. Once it blends then add the herbal tea & oil mixture and heat it all back up until it blends evenly. During this process you can add essential oils if you like. Once it cools it is ready for the jars and to be used. You can experiment with the desired thickness of the

salve by adding or subtracting the amount of wax and or butters.

To make herbal ointments, take two heaped double handfuls of your desired herb that have finely chopped. It is best to use flowers, leaves and or the plant fruit for ointments. Take a little over 1 lb of lard and heat it as the herbs are stirred in. After you have blended it all together well, then let this mixture cook at a high temperature while you are stirring until it begins to fry. At this point gradually reduce the heat and then turn it off. Let it stand overnight. The next day rewarm the concoction lightly then filter through a piece of cheesecloth and while still warm put it in your jars. You can experiment with different ingredients once again, until you get the desired product.

To make oils simply pack an empty bottle loosely with the flower or leaves of your desired herb, finely chopped, up to the neck, cold-pressed olive oil is then poured over the herbs until the oil level is about two fingers above the herbs. Let stand for 14 days in the sun or near a warm stove. Make sure it doesn't get cooked. The olive oil will draw the essence out of the herbs. After the 14 days is up, you can strain or leave the herbs in for a stronger oil. If you choose to leave the herbs in, use a sieve when you are ready to apply your oil.

Very few people nowadays even know what a poultice is, however they were used extensively during the early years of our country by the Indians and settlers. My mother taught us how to make them because she used them on us as kids, when we got any chest congestion. A poultice is an application of any moisten substance applied to a cloth and used to administer a remedy to an area of the skin. It can be used to soothe, to irritate , or to draw impurities from an area, depending on which plants or plant parts are used. The herbs used in a poultice need to be pulverized or finely chopped so that the plant is bruised. Put this substance in a sieve and hang that sieve over a boiling pot of water. While the herb is still hot, spread the mass on a piece of cloth and apply it directly over the target area as hot as the patient can stand it. Wrap several layers of cloth around this area and make sure that it stays moist by using hot water periodically. Keep the area covered for at least two to three hours or overnight if necessary. One type of poultice my mother use to make was a mustard poultice for all my siblings when we had any congestion and it would clear up overnight.

I mentioned in a previous chapter that I would outlined the procedure for giving yourself or someone else a high enema. Before I do so, I need to list some food items that can be used to flush the intestinal tract for those who need cleansing, but are not partial to enemas. Most people frown on enemas, however they are very effective and crucial in some cases. A colonic is the best and most thorough way to cleanse the intestinal tract, then the enema, then colon cleansing herbal formulas and laxative foods, in that descending order of effectiveness. Following is a list of laxative foods:

Prunes	Celery
Dates	Lettuce
Figs	Okra
Oranges	Onions
Apples	Agar-agar
Bananas	Turnips
Pears	Squash
Peaches	Parsnips

Grapes	Carrots
Grapefruits	Olives
Watermelons	Olive Oil
Lemons	Walnuts
Raisins	Butternuts
Bran	Cauliflower
Bran Muffins	Pumpkin
Bran Bread	Blueberries
Whole Grain Bread	Cherries
Spinach	

Stay away from the following constipation foods:

White Bread	Boiled Milk
White Rice	Hard Boiled Eggs
Barley	Meat
Blackberries	Cheese

HIGH ENEMA TECHNIQUE

Boil 4 quarts of distilled, purified or spring water then add 6 Tablespoons of organic coffee and let simmer. After the mixture has cooled, it can be strained. To make sure the temperature is correct , pour a little on the back of your hand. It shouldn't be too hot for your hand. Remember your body temperature is around 98 degrees. You want it warm enough, but not so cold that it will be unpleasant, nor too hot to injure yourself. You will need an enema kit which will come with an enema bag or can and the water tubing with insertion tip. When an adult is healthy and their colon clean, they should be able to retain 4 quarts of fluid before expelling it. However, to start with try to hold 1-2 quarts for 15 minutes. Before you start, allow a little fluid to flow through the tube and exit, then shut off the flow.

This is done to expel all the air, so you want have air bubbles in your colon. By laying on your side, left side preferably, insert the tip after lubricating it with vitamin E oil, olive or coconut oil, into the rectum gently. Allow the fluid to flow slowly into your colon. You may turn on your other side or change position to your back to allow more water to enter. When you feel full, remove the tip and try to retain the fluid for 15 minutes before relieving yourself. Depending on how much waste exits your system, you may want to repeat the process until only clear liquid is expelled. The reason you should change positions and hold the fluid, is to allow the liquid to travel into all the pockets and folds of the intestine. The reason organic coffee is suggested is because it has a stimulating effect on the liver causing it to throw off toxins. The caffeine has no side effect on the body when taken in this manner. Aside from coffee, you can use various herbs like Slippery elm, Chamomile, Black Walnut Hulls, Cascara Sagrada and Senna Leaves, all made into teas. You can use a solution of Sea Salt and water, Hydrogen Peroxide or plain distilled water also. Another wonderful solution that may be as effective as organic coffee is a solution of water and bicarbonate soda or sodium bicarbonate because of the sodas healing properties mentioned in the chapter on cancers. You can use about the same amount of bicarbonate soda as organic coffee in your solution. While you are detoxing or juicing you should cleanse yourself every 2-3 days at least. After you have detoxed, you should not need to take an enema for several months or so. Some people take them monthly, however a few times a year should keep your system clean, especially if you change your eating habits. It really depends on your diet. If you eat primarily fruits, vegetables, grains, seeds and little meat, you should not need to take more than 3-4 enemas a year, if that many.

In conclusion I just want to say, I realize that most of this information may never be used by the average person. There will always be someone desperate enough to take the initiative and spend the time and energy to assist their bodies in healing, regardless of the difficulties. It will depend on whether they are sick enough of being sick, to make some changes. There will always be those who will just die rather than make any changes. I enjoy life and I will always want to learn more to better my existence so I can be a greater blessing to my family and to others. It all boils down to your individual determination to be the best you can be, at any cost. If you incorporate some of these techniques into your life, you can walk in divine health and not need a doctor!

Key points outlined in chapter

(1)

(2)

(3)

(4)

(5)

Changes I can make to improve my health

(1)

(2)

(3)

(4)

(5)

CHAPTER THIRTEEN
THE TRUTH YOU KNOW WILL SET YOU FREE

It is time for you to make some decisions unless you have already done so. I have endeavored to give you enough vital information to make a quality decision concerning your food choices and healthcare concerns. I have given you the facts in regards to the health crisis in our country and I have presented you with some healthy alternatives. What will you do with the information you have received? It has been said that there are only three types of people in the world – the Wills', the Won'ts' and the Can'ts'. Which are you? I have also tried to educate you on how the system was designed to work, pointed out some of the reasons why our systems have failed and what can be done to reverse the curse. We in the body of Christ are living far below our intended position in Christ. We should be doing better than the world because we are not of this world and the

Bible says that ...we can do all things through Christ who strengthens us!!

Gods' Word says in Ezel. 47:12, "… and the fruit thereof shall be for meat, and the leaf thereof for medicine". The Bible says in Hosea 4:6, "My people are destroyed for a lack of knowledge". "The thief comes but to kill, steal and destroy". In John 8:32, the Word of God says "And ye shall know the truth, and the truth shall make you free." We discussed earlier that to know, means to have experienced or done something. Therefore you will need to apply the knowledge you have just received in order to test its' validity and reap the rewards. Remember Jesus said that, "the prince of this world cometh", and He was referring to satan. John 14:30 Satan is daily trying to coerce you into making bad choices and decisions about your health. Jesus said that, "ye are not of the world". John 15:19. In light of these biblical verses and the fact that God can not lie, we should know without a shadow of a doubt that God has redeemed us from sickness and disease.

We need to find our joy in the Lord and not in our food. We need to eat to live and not live to eat and let the joy of the Lord be our strength. Ask God to assist you with your eating problems, so you don't open the door for satan to attack your health with sickness and disease. We can unknowingly open doors that can lead to attacks, however when you discover a truth, you must act on it. Watch what you eat and watch what you take. Remember also that doctors are practicing medicine, which means they may not always know the right thing to do or the right medicine to prescribe. How important is that fact? Your very life might depend on it! Take control of your own health by making wiser choices, read your labels and add more fruits and vegetables to your diet. Complacency is said to be the enemy of achievement and a famous author once said, "99% of failure comes from people who make excuses on a regular basis."

I didn't discuss this subject in the book, but within the last couple of years, GMO food items have been introduced into the consumer market. GMOs' are genetically modified foods or cloned foods. If you purchase any of your foods at the traditional supermarkets, then you have eaten genetically modified foods. That would include most Americans. GMO foods do not have to be labeled as such!!! The FDA is allowing those food items to be sold and consumed without the public's knowledge!!! It is all legal. Not even the so-called experts or scientist know what the effects will be on the health of the populace long term. Only God knows. So I say again you need to make some serious decisions concerning your food choices.
When we get so caught up with the physical food that we eat, we neglect the spiritual food that we so urgently need. The Bible says if we walk in the spirit, we won't fulfill the lust of the flesh. If we flip that verse around it would read, if you walk in the flesh, you won't fulfill the desires of the spirit. Study Gal. 5. When we don't walk in the spirit, the gifts of the spirit will not be in operation in our lives. No gifts, no power and burdens will not be removed nor yokes destroyed. A few years ago, I was in my private prayer time with the Lord and I asked Him, why are the youth so violent and fearless. The Lord told me that He had to raise up a generation of warriors who would be fearless and ready to fight because the previous generations were all passive, fearful and lukewarm. This generation is ready to see a demonstration of Gods' power so they will believe. This generation has to see something before they will believe, just as the

people did in Christ' day. We witness to them but we are not allowing the Holy Spirit to demonstrate His power through us because we are too in the flesh.

History has shown us that change comes at the hand of the young people. The historic civil rights movement was spearheaded by young people willing to risk their lives for change. In South African apartheid was dismantled because of the bloodshed and death of the many young people. All across Africa and the Middle East it is the young people who are dying for what they believe. The young people have always made a difference. Look at the Israelites, the old generation died out so a fearless leader like Joshua could lead them to the promised land. When Joshua was a young man he was ready to take the land.

We need to forget about all that food we think we need, get our bodies healed then get up early every morning and spend some quality time with God, so He can trust us with His power. When we do that, the young people will see a demonstration of His power, they will get saved and filled and we will see the greatest revival we have ever seen as the young saints usher in the second coming.

I will conclude with an old Chinese saying, "disease enters through the mouth." God said, "My spirit shall not always strive with man, for he also is flesh; yet his days shall be an hundred and twenty years." Gen. 6:3 If God said it, that settles it, and I for one believe it. Be blessed!!! Don't forget my invite to your 120 year old birthday party!!!

RECIPES FOR LIFE

MOCK MEAT OR MEAT SUBSTITUTE

1 Cup of finely chopped Portabella Mushrooms
1/2 Cup of finely chopped nuts (for best flavor use four or five nuts - I use filberts, pecans, almonds, cashews and brazils)
1/2 Cup of Vegetable protein
½ Cup diced or minced onions
½ Cup of Humus (I use garlic or olive humus)
½ Cup of Israeli Cous Cous cooked
Blend all of the above ingredients in a bowl thoroughly. Next use ½ – 1 Tablespoon of Miso, blend in ½ – 1 Tablespoon of olive oil and ½ Cup of organic ketsup. After you blend these three ingredients together then add them to the mix. Continue to stir as you add pepper, garlic salt, cayenne pepper to taste and 2 Tablespoons of Trader Joes' South African Smoke blend seasoning (this will give the mock meat a slight BBQ taste). Your mock meat is complete. You can refrigerate until you need it. As it sits the flavors will continue to blend. It can be grilled or lightly fried in flaxseed or cocoanut oil or just used as a spread on sandwiches or as an addition to a salad.

MOCK TUNA

Soak 1 Cup of raw cashews and 1 Cup of raw sunflower seeds in 2 Cups of filtered water for 12 – 24 hours, then drain and rinse the mixture. Put the mixture in a food processor and process it until it is the consistency or tuna.
Remove the mixture from the food processor and put in a bowl then add your seasonings. Whatever seasonings you use in your tuna salad include in the bowl. We like minced onions, minced celery and bell pepper. We then add salt a little cumin and minced garlic or garlic power, all to taste. We make our own

mayonnaise and our recipe for mayonnaise is simple. We use 1 free range chicken egg, mustard, sea salt and avocado oil. Blend as follow: whip up your egg as though you were going to make scrambled eggs then add 1 Tablespoon of mustard, ½ teaspoon of salt and mix with a hand mixer as you slowly add avocado oil to your desired consistency. You will need from ¾ cup of oil to 1 ¼ cup depending on your taste. Make sure you add the oil very slowly as you mix to keep the blend from separating. Once your mayonnaise is completed, add the desired amount to your mock tuna blend, refrigerate and serve.

SEAWEED APPETIZERS

From your local supermarket, usually in the Asian, Japanese or International Foods section, you should find Seaweed Wraps in several shapes and sizes. You will want to purchase the small size, used often for sushi rolls.
I like to take the wraps and add the following item:
2 diced olives green or black, 1 heaping teaspoon of my favorite humus, 2 teaspoons of cooked brown rice or Israeli couscous, 1 teaspoon of minced onions and 1 teaspoon of diced tomatoes – roll up tightly and enjoy. I personally make only about 2 at a time because I don't like mine to get soggy!
These are some variations of the above recipe.
Use the mock meat and a leaf of lettuce or cabbage and roll up!
Use the mock tuna with some feta cheese and a little Miso then roll up!
Be creative and enjoy your new way of eating. You will work a little harder but the health improvements will be worth it!

Another variation of the above recipes is to use egg rolls instead of seaweed for your wrap. You can find the egg roll dough already cut and prepared in the refrigerated section of your supermarket. Stuff your favorite foods in the rolls, fold, brush with olive oil and lightly grill. Seaweed is healthier!!

SALAD DRESSINGS

Once you start eating healthy, you will find that you eat a lot of salads and you will make up your own salad recipes. Nothing sets a salad off more than the right dressing. I will give you the recipes for some of our favorite dressings.

Avocado Dressing

Mash the pulp of one medium size avocado. Add the juice from ½ of an orange and ½ of a lemon gradually. Whip it up until it has a smooth creamy consistency. Add some honey to taste if you are eating a fruit salad or add some finely minced onion if used on a vegetable salad.

French Dressing

Combine ½ cup of olive oil, ¼ cup of lemon juice, and the juice from one medium size tomato squeezed. To this mixture add pepper and sea salt to taste and blend well.

Fruit Dressing

Mix 3 Tablespoons of lemon juice and orange juice with 1 Tablespoon of honey and 4 Tablespoons of olive oil. Blend well. Can be used over a fruit salad or vegetable salad.

Herb Dressing

Combine 1 cup of olive oil with 1/3 cup lemon juice, ¼ teaspoon each of oregano, basil, thyme, minced garlic, paprika and rosemary. Mix this blend in a mixer until smooth as you add 2 Tablespoons of honey.

Humus Dressing

To my favorite humus I like to add olive oil and Liquid Amino and blend together until I get a desired consistency and taste then pour over my salads. You are only limited by the variety of humus mixtures, with this dressing.

Thick Lemon Dressing

Chop up finely 1 teaspoon of pecans and 1 teaspoon of almonds. Add 1 Tablespoon of lemon juice and mix it up well and let it stand for 15 minutes. Afterward add 2 Tablespoons of olive oil and beat until creamy. Add ½ teaspoon of caraway, aniseed or mustard seeds and continue blending. WHENEVER USING NUTS IT IS BEST TO USE RAW NUTS AND SOAK THEM 12-24 HOURS BEFORE USING, DRAIN AND RINSE. This helps with the digestion of nuts!

Tomato nut Dressing

Mix together ½ cup of tomatoes, peeled and mashed, ¼ cup of almonds or pecans, finely minced. In a mixer add the desired amount of olive oil as you blend this all together. You may add sea salt and pepper to taste.

MAIN DISHES & CASSEROLES

Mock Meat Eggplant Casserole
2 cups of mock meat
1 small spaghetti squash
1 small eggplant
1 32 oz, bottle of Puttanesco Sauce or make up your own
1 cup of organic corn
8 oz of parmesan cheese grated
6 corn tortillas
1 teaspoon each of oregano, thyme & sage
½ teaspoon of sea salt & pepper
Slice your eggplant in ¼" slices and grate your spaghetti squash. Blend all your seasonings together well. Oil the bottom of a large casserole dish with olive oil. Place 3 tortillas equally spaced and overlapping on the bottom of the dish then spoon about ½ inch of spaghetti squash over the tortillas evenly. Next put a layer of eggplant overlapping just enough to cover the dish. Sprinkle on ½ the seasoning evenly. Place a layer of cheese about ½ inch across the dish. Spread all the mock meat evenly on next then add about ½ inch of sauce spread evenly. If you use a large dish, you will be able to add a second layer repeating the process except do not add the initial 3 tortillas. After the second layer place 3 tortillas across the top evenly spaced and overlapping then bake in oven at 375 degrees for about 30 – 40 minutes. Let cool slightly then serve. This will serve 6 – 8 people.

VEGETARIAN SAUSAGE LINKS
1 small onion, 3 cloves garlic
2 cups cooked cold brown rice
1 cup cooked kidney beans

¼ cup egg substitute

½ cup of dried bread crumbs

3 tablespoons of flaxseed oil

2 tablespoons of grated parmesan cheese

1 cup minced collard greens

1 cup of warm tomato sauce

1 teaspoon each of thyme, oregano & sage

In a large nonstick frying pan, saute the onions in 1 tablespoon of the oil until soft, about 5 minutes. Add the collard greens, cheese, and garlic. Saute until the greens wilt, about 3 minutes. In a large bowl combine the rice, beans, egg substitute, thyme, oregano, and sage. Stir in the onion mixture. Transfer to a food processor. Process just until the mixture is a solid mass but not pureed, about 6 seconds. Divide into eight parts. Form each part into a sausage shape. Roll in the bread crumbs. Coat a baking sheet with nonstick spray. Set the sausages on the sheet and brush with the remaining oil. Broil until mottled brown on all sides, about 5 or 6 minutes. Serves 4 people.

ENCHILADAS with CHEESE and KALE

2 cups shredded kale

½ cup minced scallions

1 cup shredded low-fat Monterey Jack cheese or soy cheese

1 cup salsa

8 corn tortillas

2 tablespoons flaxseed oil

In a large nonstick frying pan over medium heat, saute the kale and scallions in 1 tablespoon of oil until tender, about 5 minutes. Divide the mixture among the tortillas. Top with the cheese. Roll up each tortilla to enclose the filling. Clean the frying pan and warm it over medium heat. Add the remaining 1 tablespoon oil. Place the enchiladas, seam-side down, in the pan.

Let brown for several minutes on each side. Add the salsa. Cover the pan, reduce the heat and simmer for about 5 minutes, basting frequently. Let stand then serve. You may add eggs, mushrooms and or olives as an option.

GARLIC and EGGPLANT SALAD
1 eggplant
1 whole garlic bulb
2 onions, thinly sliced
2 sweet red peppers, sliced
2 tablespoons of flaxseed oil
1 tablespoon dried thyme
2 cups shredded collard greens
Peel the eggplant and cut into 1 – inch chunks. Blanch in boiling water until just tender, about 4 minutes. Drain and pat dry. Separate the garlic bulb into cloves and peel each. In a 9x13-inch glass baking dish, combine the eggplant, garlic, onions, peppers, oil, and thyme. Stir to coat the vegetables with the oil. Bake uncovered at 450 degrees F until the vegetables are brown, about 25 minutes (stir a few times during cooking). Remove from the oven. Serve the vegetables warm or at room temperature on a bed of collards. Eat with the bread croutons (optional) or serve with homemade crackers. Serves 4 people

SALMON SALAD with ALMONDS and BOK CHOY
8 oz cooked salmon
2 cups sliced bok choy
¼ cup sliced almonds
2 scallions minced
1 cup nonfat yogurt
2 tablespoons crumbled blue cheese
Break the salmon into bite-size chunks. Place in a large bowl.

Add the bok choy, almonds, and scallions. In a small bowl, combine the yogurt and cheese. Combine with the salmon mixture. Serves 4 people

FOUR GRAIN KALE with LAMB CHOPS
2 medium size lamb chops – 1" thick
4 cups of fresh kale shredded
2 tablespoons dried millet
2 tablespoons dried buckwheat
2 tablespoons dried amaranth
2 tablespoons dried quinoa
1 medium size onion chopped
8 oz of mushrooms
3 tablespoons of olive oil
½ teaspoon each of garlic salt, pepper, cumin, sea salt
1 tablespoon of Trader's Joes So. African Smoke seasoning blend
2 teaspoons of Liquid Aminos (Braggs')
4 cups water

In a sauce pan rinse and boil the millet, buckwheat, amaranth and quinoa in about 4 cups of water, After it boils reduce the heat to a simmer and cover until grains are tender and water has been soaked up. Put 1 tablespoon of oil in the bottom of the crock pot. Put the crock pot on low and let it warm as you season both sides of the lamb chops with the sea salt, garlic salt, pepper, cumin and Smoke blend. Place chops in the crock pot and let cook for 3 hours on low. After 3 hours take lamb chop out and place them in a covered dish. Add the cooked grains to the liquid in the crock pot. Place the lamb chops over the grain and let cook about 10 minutes. While that is cooking saute the kale, mushrooms and onions in a skillet with 2 tablespoons of olive oil. Add the Liquid Aminos to the saute as you stir. Place your lamb chops on a plate then scoop out the grains and cover with the sauteed vegetables. (Buckwheat, amaranth and quinoa are actually seeds not grains)

DELICIOUS SOUPS

LUSCIOUS POTATO SOUP
2 cups chopped onions
1 cup diced carrots
1 cup chopped celery
6 medium potatoes diced
1 quart stock (use 2 cups each of fresh spinach & romaine lettuce juice)
1 ½ cups of almond milk
¼ cup flaxseed oil
1 teaspoon each of marjoram, dill & caraway seeds
2 teaspoons of sea salt
½ teaspoon of paprika
Heat the oil in a pressure cooker or large soup pot; saute the onions, carrots, celery, and potatoes until the onions are transparent. Pour in the stock, sea salt, spices, and milk, bring to a boil, cover and pressure cook for 20 minutes, or simmer about 1 hour until the potatoes are very tender, but won't fall apart. Serve hot with favorite toast.

CURRIED GARBANZO SOUP
½ cup dried garbanzos, cooked tender
4 cups stock (1 ½ cups each of kale & spinach juice, 1/4 cup romaine lettuce juice, ¼ cup of cilantro juice, and ¼ cup of bell pepper juice)

1 large carrot, sliced small
1 stalk celery, chopped
¼ cup almond milk
1 teaspoon curry powder
salt & pepper to taste
Heat the stock, then remove a small amount, enough to puree the garbanzos. Buzz the beans in a blender, then add them to the pot. Sprinkle in the curry, and add the milk. Bring the soup to a boil; add the celery and carrots. Simmer the soup until the vegetables are tender but not mushy. Serve hot, or try it cold if there is any left over.

CASHEW and CARROT SOUP
1 cup raw cashew pieces or chopped whole cashews
1/3 cup raw brown rice
1 cup raisins
1 cup chopped apples
1 ½ cups chopped onions
2 ½ cups almond milk
3 ounces tomato paste
¼ cup flaxseed oil
1-3 teaspoons honey (optional)
4 cups grated carrots packed
1 tablespoon butter
2 teaspoons sea salt
6 cups of stock (2 cups each of spinach & kale juice, 1 cup romaine lettuce juice, and ½ cup each cilantro & bell pepper juice)
Melt the butter and add oil to a soup pot or pressure cooker; saute the chopped onions for 1 minute, stir in carrots and saute until the onions are soft and transparent. They will be orange rather than brown. Stir in the tomato paste, apple, stock, and

salt. Bring the mixture to a boil and stir in the brown rice. Cover and pressure cook for 15 minutes, or cook regularly for about 45 minutes, until the soup is a beautiful orange and the carrots are tender, but not mushy. Add the raisins and cashew and optional honey, bring to a boil again, and simmer until the raisins are plump – about 5 minutes. Add the milk and heat thoroughly.

HEARTY CABBAGE SOUP
8 CUPS OF STOCK (2 cups each of spinach, romaine lettuce & kale juice, ½ cup each of onion, carrot, cilantro & bell pepper juice)
7 – 8 cups of shredded cabbage into ¾ inch pieces (about 2 lbs.)
2 ½ cups of diced potatoes
3 – 4 chopped tomatoes
2 ½ cups yogurt (optional)
1 ½ cups chopped onions
1 cup of chopped carrots
½ – 1 cup tomato sauce
¼ – ½ cup chopped fresh parsley
1 cup chopped celery
½ cup dry kidney beans
3/4 cup raw brown rice, cooked
½ cup cous cous, cooked
¼ cup flaxseed oil
2 teaspoons minced garlic
1 bay leaf
1 teaspoon of thyme
sea salt to taste
Heat the oil in a large soup pot or dutch oven; saute the onions, carrots, celery, and potatoes for about 10 minutes, until the

onions are soft and transparent and the potatoes are translucent. Add a little oil and stir in the cabbage; saute until the cabbage is soft and its volume is reduced. Stir in the stock, all the seasonings, plus the kidney beans, cous cous, and rice. Bring the mixture to a boil, lower the heat, cover, and simmer about ½ hour. Just before you serve, stir in the chopped tomatoes. Top each cup with ¼ cup of yogurt (or use 2 tablespoons of grated cheese or cottage cheese).

HOT CHEESE SOUP
5 cups of stock (2 cups each of spinach & kale juice, ½ cup of romaine lettuce and ¼ cup each of cilantro & bell pepper juice)
½ lb of cheddar (or soft cheese), grated -about 2 cups
1 ¼ cups toasted sunflower seeds
½ cup sesame tahini or sesame butter, 1/4 cup flour
¼ cup each of finely chopped carrots & celery
¼ cup minced onion
¼ cup finely chopped red sweet pepper
2 tablespoons minced hot green chili peppers
2 tablespoons butter
6 tablespoons almond milk
1 teaspoon sea salt
Melt the butter in a large soup pot; saute the onions, red pepper, and hot pepper until all vegetables are soft, but not brown. Stir in the flour and heat for 1 minute; add the stock and bring the mixture to a boil. Use a whisk to blend in the tahini (which will look curdled). Lower the heat and simmer for five minutes. Add the cheese by handfuls, whisking until each one has melted completely. Add the milk. Add the salt, and just before serving, stir in the sunflowers. Use whatever flour you desire.

REFERENCES AND SUGGESTED READING

BACK TO EDEN by Jethro Kloss

BEFORE YOU CALL THE DOCTOR – Safe, Effective Self-Care for Over 300 Common Medical Problems by Dr. Anne Simons, Bobbie Hasselbring and Michael Castleman

ENZYME NUTRITION by Dr. Edward Howell

EVERYBODY'S GUIDE TO HOMEOPATHIC MEDICINES by Dr. Stephen Cummings and Dana Ullman, m.p.h.

FRUITS, VEGETABLES AND HERBS by Heinerman

HEALTH THROUGH GOD'S PHARMACY by Maria Treben

HOW TO GET RID OF POISONS IN YOUR BODY by Gary Null and Steven Null

INTRODUCTION TO NATURAL HEALTH by Dr. Terrence Leon Sullivan

NATURAL HEALTH REMEDIES by Janet Maccaro, PH. D., C.N.C.

NUTRITION AND MENTAL ILLNESS – An Orthomolecular Approach to Balancing Body Chemistry by Carl C. Pfeiffer PH.D., M.D.

NATURAL DIET FOR FOLKS WHO EAT – Cooking with Mother Nature by Dick Gregory

PRESCRIPTION FOR NUTRITIONAL HEALING by Dr. James F. Balch and Phyllis A. Balch, C.N.C.

RECIPES FOR A SMALL PLANET by Ellen Buchman Ewald

REDISCOVER THE KINGDOM by Dr. Myles Monroe
THE CAUSE OF DISEASE IN AMERICA by Dr. Terrence
Leon Sullivan

THE GERSON THERAPY by Charlotte Gerson D.P.M. And
Morton Walker D.P.M.

THE GOOD FOOD REVOLUTION by Will Allen with
Charles Wilson

THE HEALING FOODS COOKBOOK by The Prevention
Magazine Editors

THE HERB BOOK by John Lust

THE HOLY BIBLE KJV, NKJV, MESSAGE VERSION AND
THE AMPLIFIED

THE WILDFOOD TRAILGUIDE by Allan Hall

3 HIDDEN WAYS WHEAT MAKES YOU FAT by Dr. Mark
Hyman

WHEAT BELLY – LOSE THE WHEAT, LOSE THE WEIGHT,
and Find your Path to Health by Dr. William Davis

WHO SWITCHED OFF MY BRAIN? - Controlling Toxic
Thoughts and Emotions by Caroline Leaf

ACKNOWLEDGEMENT

I would like to acknowledge and thank the following people for assisting me with the completion of this project. To Gloria Bush, who is active also in the natural health field, I would like to thank you for your editing skills and corrections. To my pastor, Senior pastor and founder of Antelope Valley Christian Center, Tom Pickens for your inspiration to complete this book with your recent message on "Passion" and your time and expertise in reviewing the project for scriptural integrity, I thank you and appreciate your leadership. To my loving son Jeff Burns, for assistance in doing the whole project with your computer skills and publishing incite, not to mention your awesome cover design and layout, I am so grateful. Finally to my wife, who has been with me through the entire health journey as we together have incorporated these principles into our lives, I can't communicate how much I love and appreciate you, my better half!!!

To my Lord and Savior, Jesus Christ, The Father and my helper The Holy Spirit I thank you for making all things possible and for loving and caring for me.

SALVATION PRAYER

GOD IS A SPIRIT AND THOSE THAT WORSHIP HIM AND WANT TO KNOW HIM MUST BE BORN OF THAT SAME SPIRIT. WE HUMAN BEINGS ARE SPIRITS MADE BY GOD WITH BODIES AND SOULS WHICH ARE COMPOSED OF MIND, WILL, EMOTION, INTELLECT AND IMAGINATION. OUR SPIRITS, WHICH ARE THE REAL PERSON HAVE BEEN SEPARATED FROM GOD BY SIN. WE WERE ALL BORN SINNERS IN NEED OF SALVATION. ONLY THROUGH THE ACCEPTANCE OF THE PERFECT SACRIFICE, WHICH IS GOD'S ONLY SON JESUS CHRIST, CAN WE BE REUNITED WITH OUR FATHER GOD. TO FULLY UNDERSTAND THE CONTENT OF THIS BOOK AND TO MORE IMPORTANTLY UNDERSTAND GOD'S WORD THE HOLY BIBLE, WHICH IS HIS WILL, WE NEED TO MAKE THE DECISION TO ACCEPT JESUS CHRIST AS OUR OWN PERSONAL SAVIOR. HIS WORDS ARE SPIRIT AND LIFE. BY REPEATING THE FOLLOWING PRAYER WITH SINCERITY OF HEART, YOU TO CAN OBTAIN ETERNAL LIFE WITH GOD IN HEAVEN AND AVOID ETERNAL LIFE IN HELL WITH SATAN. This prayer has nothing whatsoever to do with religion or membership in any physical church, it only involves your personal relationship with the GOD that created you!

SAY: DEAR GOD IN HEAVEN I AM A SINNER IN NEED OF A SAVIOR AND I BELIEVE THAT YOUR ONLY SON JESUS CHRIST WAS BORN, DIED AND WAS RESURRECTED FOR MY SINS. I RECEIVE HIM NOW AS MY PERSONAL LORD AND SAVIOR AND I THANK YOU THAT I AM UNITED WITH YOU AND A MEMBER OF

YOUR BODY. I THANK YOU THAT ALL MY SINS HAVE BEEN FORGIVEN AND I AM IN PERFECT STANDING WITH YOU, A NEW CREATION. FILL ME WITH YOUR PRECIOUS HOLY SPIRIT SO I MAY LIVE A LIFE PLEASING TO YOU AND RECEIVE ALL YOUR PRECIOUS PROMISES. I PRAY THIS AND I THANK YOU IN JESUS NAME AMEN!

If you just prayed this prayer for the first time, let us know. You are now saved and filled with the Holy Spirit and a possessor of eternal life with God!!

EMAIL thewordnaction@gmail.com

CONTACT

If you need to correspond with Minister Burns for any reason including, Book signings, workshops, seminars, lectures or interviews please use the following contact information:
Minister Leonard F. Burns
EMAIL thewordnaction@gmail.com
May you and your loved ones enjoy Divine Health
in Jesus name, Amen!!!

For additional copies of this book visit Amazon.com, Bookstores and Online Retailers.

Made in the USA
Charleston, SC
06 February 2013